RAISING A CHILD
RESPONSIBLY
IN A SEXUALLY
PERMISSIVE WORLD

D0106924

RAISING A CHILD RESPONSIBLY IN A SEXUALLY PERMISSIVE WORLD

Sol Gordon, Ph.D., Judith Gordon, M.S.W.

Adams Media Corporation
Holbrook, Massachusetts

Published by
Adams Media Corporation
260 Center Street, Holbrook, MA 02343

ISBN: 1-58062-177-5

Printed in the United States of America

JIHGFEDCB

This book was originally published as *Raising a Child Conservatively
in a Sexually Permissive World* by Sol Gordon and Judith Gordon in 1989
by Fireside, a division of Simon & Schuster.

Library of Congress Cataloging-in-Publication Data
available from publisher.

Cover photo by Bluestone Productions (FPG International)

Visit our home page at http://www.adamsmedia.com

In loving memory
of Dr. Mary S. Calderone,
my friend and mentor

1904–1998

"Doctor Challenged 'Sexophobic' Society"
Headline in Associated Press obituary, Oct. 25, 1998

CONTENTS

Preface ix

P R E F A C E

I

The "we" of this 1999 revision of our book is the undying spirit and sensitivity of my late wife Judith—to whom this edition is dedicated. Sharing the honor are Diana and Norman Fleishman, wonderful human beings, askable parents, and my good friends who are responsible for much of the creative ideas which greatly enhance our new work. In the spirit again of my Danish wife, I say, "Tak for alt."

II

If there are five critical messages that we would offer parents— more significant than the "facts about sex"—to help boost self-esteem and responsibility, they would be these:

1. Parents are the main sex educators of their children, whether they like it or not—whether they want to be or not.
2. Parents, if they want to be "askable," must be prepared for any question or incident that involves their children's sexuality. One good way—in response to any question, however embarrassing—is for parents to respond by saying, "That's a good question." Answer on the spot or say, "We'll discuss it when we get home." If your child "catches" you reading this book, use it as an opportunity to share with them an appropriate passage.

3. Somehow get across to your children that nothing that ever happens to them will be made worse by talking to you about it. We've got to open up communication.
4. Children are not perfect. They make mistakes, and it's up to us to turn their mistakes into lessons.
5. And, finally, failure is an event—*not* a person. Children who are loved grow into adults who like themselves. They don't exploit others, and are not likely to be exploited.

—August 1999

CHAPTER ONE

The Family and the "Sexual Revolution"

W e as a society are good at discussing and declaring our morality, but we find it hard to face up to the consequences of our behavior. Many of us have lived through the assassinations of the sixties and seventies, and Vietnam, and we are still witnessing the deterioration of our cities due to neglect and crime. Most of us—at least those who have not been directly victimized by these forces and events—have not been affected in our daily lives: we have moved away, accommodated, forgotten, repressed.

We are more preoccupied with our private lives and our families, primarily with protecting and enjoying our children. Yet, more than 50 percent of all U.S. marriages end in divorce; about 70 percent of adolescents will engage in sexual intercourse before they graduate from high school. There are 1.3 million pregnancies each year among girls before their twentieth birthday, as well as several million new cases of venereal disease. Then there is the accepted fact that the majority of men and women engage in premarital and/or extramarital sexual relations. The National Center for Health Statistics reports that the birth rate among teenagers was 56.8 per thousand in 1995. The birth rate in the United States is now twice as high as in England and Wales or Canada and nine times as high as in the Netherlands or Japan, according to the Alan Guttmacher Institute, 1996.[1]

Our chief concern here is not hypocrisy. There is a colossal gap between what we want for ourselves and our children and what we have. We, the authors of this book, are concerned about what is going on in the average American family. We would like to be of some assistance in the crucial area of human sexuality. We have written this book not to save the world, but to convey a few basic messages. We want to help families who are trying to raise morally responsible children in this permissive world. We would like families to enjoy a sense of each other, parents to trust their children, and children to confide in their parents.

It is common to read that our world has become a less safe place for children because of a "sexual revolution," a new morality whose main ethic is "Everyone should be free from repression and should do his or her own thing," or, simply, "If it feels good, do it." We live with a drumbeat of TV ads hawking immediate gratification. The masters of manipulation target us every two minutes, now, to exchange their cure-alls for being loved, for removing our loneliness, anxiety, fear, and gloom—in exchange for our cash. They offer one solution: "Buy!" and one philosophy: "You are what you own." It is in this environment that our children are growing up, not the one in which their parents were raised. It is a world we, as those parents, seem to have little control over, despite the wish to influence it in some substantive way. It is the same world we sexuality educators deplore, however much some people hold us responsible for having caused it all.

For starters, there's television. Perhaps you have become tired of hearing about all the rape, violence, and promiscuity on prime

---

1. The pregnancy rate for single women has continued to increase. About 32.6 percent of births in 1994 were to single mothers (U.S. Census Bureau).

time. Yet there is a challenge here we cannot ignore. Years ago Benjamin Stein, a social commentator, wrote in *TV Guide*: "There is not one show on television today that's set in the present and that's not science fiction that presents a woman with young children who is married, secure and happy." Today his words still ring true. Daytime TV, too, is full of unhappy adults with unsatisfactory sex lives. Though children are usually at school during the soaps, when they are home they are bombarded by the promos. For example, a promo for *Days of Our Lives* features a glamorous woman standing before a well-dressed man; she rips off her dress, revealing a skimpy bra and panties. Then she says, "Let's play doctor!...How can you say 'no' to an offer like this?" All in 15 seconds!

Our children are further influenced by peer group pressure, fashions, "sexploitive" commercials, rock music (do it, do it), alcohol and drugs, to say nothing of the current wave of trashy films geared explicitly to teenagers.

Parents are rightly concerned over what their role should be in all this. There are so many dilemmas along the way. Parents want their children to be happy and popular. They want to nourish their children, to see them have friends and function well in school. They want their children to be moral and responsible, yet not be regarded as weird or out of the mainstream of their peer group.

How are parents to respond individually to the criticism often made that most children these days are no longer reared, they are turned loose? How do "conservative parents" respond to an outwardly permissive society?

What do we mean by conservative parents? We are not talking about the political scene, which is confusing enough. Some people regard anyone who is against prayer in the schools as a liberal. Well, we are frankly sick and tired of the political preachers across the country telling us as citizens that if we wanted to be a moral person we must believe in a certain way. There are many people and organizations who have preempted the meaning not only of conservatism, but also of family, flag, and God;

their interpretations are not shared by most true conservatives, either politically or personally.

We are broadly defining conservative families as those who love their country and respect its Constitution and laws, regardless of political affiliation, and most of whom believe in God and the Golden Rule—though they may belong to many different religions. Conservative families favor gradual as opposed to revolutionary changes to improve society. Conservatives support private enterprise (though they may draw the line at the behavior of some out-of-control multinationals who perfect the practice of "corporate welfare"). They abhor bigotry and racism and support applying the law equally. They believe that the family unit is the central constituent of this society, yet they accept the message that all human beings are worthy and precious, whatever their social status. Conservative families do not meddle in others' lives except when called upon to help. They take pride in their neighborhoods and enjoy being good neighbors. They do not want to impose their religious or moral views on others, although they are glad to share their beliefs. Conservatives differ on a wide range of issues, such as nuclear proliferation, excessive corporate subsidies, and government spending, but they generally agree that our democratic system is the best choice.

Conservative parents know, in a world where sex dominates TV, films, and music for our youth, that sexuality education is needed in the schools. They also know that teachers in this area must be well trained and respect parents' values. Most of us are opposed to censorship, and all of us are opposed to minors having access to pornography and being sexually exploited by anyone. The Internet has brought this into millions of homes, and thus we need even more knowledge, education, preparation, and prevention. And, finally, if conservatives could live according to their best aspirations, they would prefer to live and let live.

This book is about what parents can do to help guide their children and to raise them to be young adults with good self-esteem and sound values. We don't endorse repression, rash judgments motivated by fear, or abolishing the separation of church and state as acceptable means to that end. We have seen in the past few years religious fervor and hatred creating genocide and tearing countries apart. It's so important that religions come together as "one human family" to solve the enormous problems that exist. As William James, the great philosopher, said to his grandson's question about life's purpose: "There are just three things to remember: 1) Be kind; 2) Be kind; and 3) Be kind."

Parents understandably have a stake in wanting their children to adopt their own religious orientation. This is often the case in homes where children are raised to have substantial self-esteem, a healthy attitude toward their own sexuality, and trust in other people. Young people who receive from their parents the essential religious and moral messages concerning sexuality will tend to incorporate them into their sexual decision-making. Religion can also provide education and instruction in how to handle intimate relationships, as well as some of the more factual aspects of sexuality. Some churches and synagogues have already developed good programs in this area. But let us be realistic. Most churches and synagogues are having a difficult time. They must compete for attention with the mass media, chiefly television (watched by children approximately six hours a day on average). These shows and ads are created by some of the brightest, highest-paid writers on earth. (On the other hand, it has become standard in some circles to blame secular humanism for the decline of morality and spiritual observance. Our view is that organized religion must accept the responsibility for its failure to be attractive, especially to young people.)

Ironically, sexuality, including the physical and psychic pleasure it provides, has been the source of great anxiety and controversy. The association of sex with the Fall of Mankind, and the resulting burdens of sin and guilt, colors many people's attitudes toward their own sexuality. The human conscience has always wrestled with these moral issues. As a result, many religious educators rely on abstinence alone in their sexuality education, which completely ignores the reality of today's world and contemporary teenage behavior.

For those who find little meaning in religion itself, sexuality has spiritual connotations that need not be identified with any religious denomination or persuasion. As Abraham Maslow points out in his book *Religious Values and Peak Experiences*,[2] "[S]piritual values do not need supernatural concepts to support them."

Some readers will suspect that while we claim to be conservative, our views concerning sexuality are hardly so. This is, of course, their privilege, but we ask our readers for a larger understanding. Sexuality is, after all, a sensitive subject, and an all-too-common reading of the conservative position implies an opposition to communicating about sexuality, either at home or in churches and schools. Some people, therefore, might feel that our advocacy of communication between parent and child disqualifies us as conservatives, or even that it indicts us as part of the permissive society we're concerned with. It is the quality of such communication that distinguishes us as conservative. We advocate mature, educational discussions that are mindful of morals and responsibility.

Even we were astonished by the response of our college students who were given the assignment of discussing two of our children's books with their parents—*Did the Sun Shine Before You Were Born?*, designed for children under six years of age, and *Girls Are Girls and Boys Are Boys—So What's the Difference?*, for children aged six to nine. We received reports from more than a thousand students; most of their parents, the majority of whom were college-educated, revealed that they would have been uncomfortable letting their children read these books at the appropriate ages. Some would have refused. Yet, most also admitted that they

---

2. A Penguin publication, 1970.

would allow the same appropriately aged children to read them now. It seems that the events of the intervening years (including the huge increase in the use of sex to sell programs, products, and news) have influenced them.

Following are several excerpts from the students' project:

Overall, I enjoyed doing this assignment. I was shocked that my parents felt so positively about it [the book]. Before undertaking this project, I felt that they would be totally against giving a book like this to small children.

Although they never utilized any kind of formal education with their children, both of my parents said that they would have felt comfortable using the book as a teaching aid, but that they would not want the book to be within reach of a young child. They felt that *Girls Are Girls*...must be read with an adult on hand, in order to explain, expand, discuss and answer any questions the child might have. My parents' reaction to the book surprised me. Because of my lack of formal sex education at home, I assumed the subject made them uncomfortable and was taboo.

My parents do not feel that this book is suitable for any age group. Both of them believe that sex education should not begin until puberty, and that this book would be superficial at that time.

The best part of this assignment was the fact that it gave me the opportunity to have a meaningful sex-oriented conversation with my parents. Not only did we discuss *Girls Are Girls*...but we also talked about such things as premarital sex, birth control and abortion. My parents were uncomfortable talking about these things but said later they were glad we had—and wished we had started sooner.

The real benefit of this assignment for our students, despite initial apprehension, was that they felt enthusiastic about it afterward. Though some of the parents were reluctant to begin, the books stimulated one of the few—if not the only—discussions the students had ever had with their parents about sexuality. The assignment served to underscore the statistic that less than 20 percent of parents ever have significant discussions with their children about sex (the typical one-shot mother–daughter talks about menstruation notwithstanding).

We do appreciate that sexuality is a difficult subject for many parents, yet a bumper sticker sighted the other day makes great sense to us: "If you think education is costly, try ignorance." A recurring theme in this book is, don't operate on the assumption that young people know everything these days. Where are they getting their knowledge? From parents? From the schools? From churches and synagogues? No, most of what young people know they get from one another, videos, CDs, films, and TV, and most of that is just plain wrong.

Our other message states that parents are the principal sexuality educators of their children whether they like it or not, so they might as well do the best job they can. Conservative parents have much to question and criticize in our permissive society, whose chief sexual flaws are readily recognizable:

1. People have sex first and then consider getting to know each other. More often than not it's too late; the relationship is finished the morning after. It's as if the old fairy tale of the frog and the Princess had been rewritten. The modern tale is, the Princess kisses the Prince; he turns into a frog and hops away.
2. There is failure to understand that people get hurt not because they don't know how to make love, but because they don't feel loved (read Masters and Johnson's book *The Pleasure Bond*).
3. People use sex as a test of love, e.g., "If you really love me, you'll have sex with me."

4. The worst, most violent, sexist, exploitive media offerings are often the most popular. Worse has already come to worse here, and we parents have to set some good examples by limiting our children's media consumption to their special shows only, perhaps even "pulling the plug" occasionally. Children love to dissect ads, and it is a good idea to do some preventive education with them about how the ads try to manipulate. Experience suggests that the more bored, passive, vulnerable, and exploitable a child is, the more that child watches television.

5. Sexuality is equated with orgasms—i.e., with physical pleasure and performance rather than with love and intimacy.

We like what the popular psychologist and author Sam Keen once said: "When our Eros is limited to genital sexuality, it becomes obsessive, and boring, and finally destructive." The so-called sexual revolution offers little comfort to millions of lonely, alienated, desperate people needing love but only "getting laid" or "scoring." Arthur Schlesinger, Jr., has suggested that if sexual repression failed to produce happiness in the nineteenth century, sexual liberation appears to have done little better in the twentieth.

Conservatives in general will applaud the *real* sexual revolution, when one's sex behavior is private, moral, responsible, and pleasurable, and when people respect each other, and lovers love each other. It will come. The question is, what do conservative parents do in the meantime?

First, become involved. A large part of this book concerns the strengthening of family life by promoting self-esteem in children. High self-esteem is correlated with growing up in families where children feel loved, valued, and that they belong. This joyful, exasperating parental task is at the cutting edge of all we believe in and write about. It can require a lot of faith on the part of parents—faith, as suggested by psychologist David C. McClelland, that loving and believing in your children will promote maturity in the long run, even if some of their behavior is unacceptable in the short run; faith that eventually they'll learn to make their own way.

Secondly, don't pine for the good old days. It's tempting to forget that in the 1930s, 25 percent of our work force was unemployed. That not long ago women and blacks couldn't vote. That only the elite went to college. And who, after all, wants to return to the irrational guilt, ignorance, and dismal repression of Victorian morality? The acclaimed psychologist Rollo May once suggested that the Victorian person sought to have love without falling into sex; the modern person seeks to have sex without falling into love.

A third step lies in recognizing that some progress has occurred. Generally speaking, parents today have the number of children they want, when they want them. Adult sex for pleasure, as opposed to sex for reproduction only, is an accepted part of life. Many physicians and health-care workers are now required to take courses in human sexuality as part of their training, something unheard of in professional schools only twenty-five years ago. Women are making progress toward being accepted and treated as equals.

Parents need to determine within their own families what to overlook and what to emphasize. This book suggests that parents should not overlook the sexuality education of their children, because no one else can take their place. Keep in mind as you read ahead that telling children only "not to" (smoke, drink, get high, have sex, or stay out late) doesn't help much unless you can also lead them to discover how to feel good about themselves. In the final analysis parents should not undertake the sexual education of their children in order to exercise ultimate control over them. Parents who do are unlikely to succeed. Rather, include sexuality education as but one part of a good relationship with your children.

This is a practical book for parents. We're keenly aware of the other problems relating to discipline of children, such as drug and alcohol abuse or performance in school, even as we address just one specific, albeit essential, aspect of child rearing. Any book that

The Family and the "Sexual Revolution"

attempts, in effect, to solve all such problems will wind up solving none of them. As the English ditty puts it: "One thing at a time and that done well/Is a very good rule as many can tell."

Nonetheless, parents who communicate with their children about the crucial topic of sexuality usually find that other areas of their relationship with their children improve as well. Psychiatrist M. Scott Peck has written, "When we desire to encourage the growth of the human spirit, we challenge and encourage the human capacity to solve problems...it is through the pain of confronting and resolving problems that we learn." With the promotion of self-esteem in our children, we will be much more likely to succeed in all of these areas.

It's not enough to feel good about yourself. Some of the meanest people we know "feel good about themselves." For us the "best" definition of self-esteem is "Appreciating my own worth and importance and having the character to be accountable for myself and to act responsibly toward others" (California State Legislative Task Force on Self-Esteem).

CHAPTER TWO

Promoting Self-Esteem in Children

P arents have the right, indeed the responsibility, to demand certain behaviors of their children, such as honesty in relationships and being trustworthy, and to forbid others, such as drugs and stealing. Yet parents must be able to distinguish between their children's behavior and the children themselves. Let's explain that. Suppose a child behaves in a way that has been forbidden—for example, he tells a lie, denying that he broke the lamp in the living room. When parents enforce appropriate discipline, it is imperative not to withdraw their love or reject the child. When scolding a child one must still convey that the child is loved and valued. The behavior itself may be bad, but the child's own sense of worth and acceptance needs to be maintained. If the parents withhold love as a punishment, the child will come to feel unloved, and unlovable. As Anne Bernstein, a well-known psychologist, has written, "Children will come to value themselves as they have been valued by the significant people in their lives: treated with respect, they will respect themselves and be respectful to others in their turn."

Let's begin with the assumption that almost all parents mean well, don't have to be perfect, and can afford to make mistakes.

13

Children appreciate it when parents acknowledge their difficulties; an implicit theme of this book is, "If you make mistakes, turn them into lessons," or even "There are no mistakes—only lessons." What is self-esteem? Children have self-esteem when they:

- Feel good about themselves;
- Trust themselves and others;
- Don't exploit anyone;
- Get along with their families;
- Have a sense of kind humor;
- Form relationships that are mutually enhancing;
- Care about other people's welfare.

A basic sense of **altruism** operates within people who feel secure enough in themselves to extend help, consideration, and respect to others. Philosopher Robert Nozick has spent his lifetime evolving a concept of the good person's development. He writes:

> The developed person will want to help perfect others; this is the most important aid he can give them. We want to find a way of living whereby our best energies and talents are poured out so as to speak to and improve the best energies and talents of others. We want to utilize our highest parts and energies in a way that helps others to flourish.[1]

This area of altruism has also been explored by Erich Fromm and Erik Erikson, among others. Viktor Frankl believes that life isn't worthwhile unless the individual possesses a sense of purpose and meaning. Hans Selye, in his pioneering work in the area of stress, found that altruism is the most significant way for people to cope with and ease the levels of stress in their daily lives. So self-esteem is not just a matter of feeling good about oneself.

---

1. Robert Nozick, *Philosophical Explanations* (Cambridge, MA: The Belknap Press of Harvard University Press, 1981, p. 513).

Yet feeling good about the self is the foundation of the kind of exemplary adulthood we describe—and that foundation is laid in childhood, in the bedrock of good parenting. A sense of basic trust is imparted in infancy itself.

A GOOD START

Generally, experts in the field of child development don't believe that it is possible to "spoil" a child in the first year of life. Parents sometimes worry that their baby will become spoiled if picked up or fed frequently, or if they respond quickly when the child cries. They fear that responsiveness will cause the child to become demanding, and to expect the same intensive attention when older. In short, parents fear that their children will become dependent and clinging. Interestingly, the opposite is usually the case. Parents who respond quickly to their crying infants and in other ways make the children feel secure will find their children becoming more **independent**. Specialists write that such children are "securely attached" to their parents; confident of their parents' love and care, they feel secure enough to explore the environment and develop their own skills.

During the first twelve months of life, then, it is better to err on the side of excess cuddling and responsiveness than on the side of minimal play and involvement with the child. This does not involve smothering the child. A prime parental challenge is not to adopt an overly rigid stance in relation to any of a child's behaviors or emotions. This crucial concept applies from birth through the child's lifetime.

In toilet-training a child, for instance, it is best to be both gentle and flexible in one's approach, and to maintain a healthy respect for the child's individual ability and readiness.[2] Weaning as well should not be harsh or abrupt and should proceed with

---

2. For example, most experts believe that toilet training should rarely start before the infant's second year. For a general parenting book, we recommend *Experts Advise Parents*, edited by Eileen Schiff, Delta Trade edition, 1988.

sensitivity to the child's psychic and physical development. Researchers have found that when this "style" of parenting is combined with warmth and nurturance toward the child, there is a greater probability that the child will in time display more comfort with all bodily processes, sexual and otherwise. There is also a greater likelihood that the child will possess confidence, high self-esteem, and an important sense of self-acceptance.

As their babies grow into curious toddlers, parents can help foster self-esteem by praising and rewarding their children for doing well. More than anything else, this helps instill a feeling of **competence**. Competence breeds faith in oneself and one's body, a belief that the world is essentially safe, and trust in other people. It also provides the child with a sense of flexibility. Children who feel competent are resilient and can bounce back from inevitable failures and disappointments, secure in the knowledge that things will work out. Dr. Thomas Gordon, author of many parenting books, including *Parent Effectiveness Training*, was asked recently by one of us, "What is the most important thing you have learned in more than 35 years in the field?" (Through Gordon Training International he educates parents, teachers, and leaders around the world.) "Punishment doesn't work, especially physical punishment, which is still used by a majority of parents," was his answer.

An issue of great concern, therefore, is that some parents interact with their children primarily around troublesome, negative situations. If parents respond to children mainly when they are crying, are in the "doghouse," are physically injured, and so on, then the pattern is repeated and many seemingly minor accomplishments may be overlooked. Saying "Good job!" or giving a hug when a child finishes a puzzle or negotiates a steep set of stairs reinforces the child's sense of competence and self-acceptance. Parents can also create positive learning experiences for their children by teaching them how to tell time, build a sand castle, tie shoes, and perform some household tasks. You can participate and have fun with your child without taking charge completely. When parents merely demonstrate for their children how to do things, the children don't get the opportunity to do for themselves. In addition, they may be left with the impression that they can never master the task as well as Mommy or Daddy does. They may also be left with a residual sense that their bodies don't work well or are somehow "wrong."

As children become verbal and start spending time with other children, it becomes especially important for them to build competence in tasks that benefit other people. Without becoming capable of being helpful to others, children may feel themselves to be of little worth. Learning how to act altruistically gives most children an important sense of purpose, which will serve them well in later life. This concept has been brilliantly elucidated by Swedish sociologist Benny Henriksson: "Never before in our history and in no other culture has it happened that people can reach the age of twenty-five without having learned to carry out a task which benefits others or without learning to take care of anyone who is old, sick, or small."

Equally important to parents is the principle of respecting the unconscious instincts and emotions of the child. Parents can impose controls and make demands gently, according to the individual child's growing ability to exercise responsibility and restraint. By not enforcing demands according to an arbitrary schedule of child development, they can enhance the child's own sense of competence. Respecting the impulse life of the child also involves accepting as valid the child's feelings and experience of the world. For instance, children often have nightmares that frighten them and awaken them in the middle of the night. Parents hurry to their bedside with reassurances that "everything's all right," and "there's nothing to worry about." Though it may be well intentioned, such advice tends to invalidate the child's feelings. A much better response would be, "You just woke up and you were really scared, weren't you? You had a scary dream. Do you want to tell me about it?...Nightmares *are* scary. Some times I have them, too. When I wake up the bad dream disappears."

Using this model, parents can enhance the child's self-understanding. Note that we are not encouraging impulsiveness in the child or a permissive attitude on the part of parents. We are saying that children's self-acceptance is bolstered when parents also accept parts of the child that may be thought of as frightening, negative, or regressive. This helps to create an atmosphere in which a wide variety of subjects are open for discussion within the family. Parents and children don't have to discuss everything—in fact, a certain degree of room for private thoughts and feelings is desirable. But this ability to communicate remains an option, especially in times of stress.

In a highly recommended book, *Your Child's Self-Esteem,* Dorothy Corille Briggs describes the inner dialogue of a child with low self-esteem: "I'm not very important. People wouldn't like me if they really knew me. I can't do things as well as others. There's not much point in my trying anything new because I know before I try that I'll fail. I can't make good decisions. I don't talk in groups because I don't say anything worth listening to. I don't like to go to new places. I hate being alone; in fact, I just wish I were someone else."

In our many years of counseling people of all ages, we have witnessed countless times how low self-esteem leaves people open to being exploited, sexually and otherwise. Such individuals believe that they deserve poor treatment; for them, even a poor relationship is better than none, and a little caring mixed with much abuse better than no caring at all. Promiscuous and exploitive sexual behavior, premature parenthood, and a range of self-damaging behaviors can easily feed off poor self-esteem.

Among people with high self-acceptance, being taken advantage of is much less likely: one's self-worth dictates that most behaviors should be in one's best interests, constructive in nature. Conservative sexual behavior in this context means that it is wisely considered, premeditated and planned for, and in harmony with the person's values. Conversely, people who don't like themselves expect to be treated according to their own evaluation—that is, poorly. They don't value their own bodies or feelings and may overly value those of other people. In this way, others are seen as good, while the self is bad and usually to blame for anything that goes wrong.

Letty Cottin Pogrebin states this in another way in her book *Growing Up Free*. She writes: "Long-term studies have found that people who are most satisfied with their bodies tend to have the most confidence, self-esteem, and satisfying sex lives."

THE MORAL ISSUE

In the emotional area of sexuality, young people, like persons of any age, can be oblivious to consequences. Here the moral dimensions of behavior and decision-making assume great importance. The child's identity is closely related to the types of decisions he or she characteristically makes, and children with high self-esteem tend to resolve problem situations in ways that benefit the self (and enhance the growth of others).

Within the boundaries of these moral considerations there is reasonable latitude for the expression of individuality. Nevertheless, parents need to draw the distinction between acceptable personal styles of moral behavior and those behaviors that are almost never acceptable. For example, there will be days on which your sixteen-year-old son may be ill-tempered and short with his girlfriend; this kind of behavior is expectable occasionally. It can be tolerated if balanced by friendliness, courtesy, and caring the rest of the time. But for your son to pressure his girlfriend to have sexual intercourse, with little regard for her feelings or no thoughts of contraception, pregnancy, or disease, is never acceptable behavior.

Moral considerations enter into political and societal forums as well. To illustrate: equality of the sexes, dignity, and respect for all human beings regardless of their race, religion, sexual orientation, or country of origin all stem from the fundamental democratic premise of equality. Equality does not always mean equal, or require identical treatment for all people all the time. People simply aren't that good or consistent. What is involved is a *striving* to be moral, despite occasional mistakes and setbacks.

Self-esteem is the cornerstone of sensible, moral decision-making. It ensures that people will not distort moral guidelines to suit their needs. Initiating a dialogue with one's children about moral issues, early in life, is necessary if they are to develop an understanding of morality. Such communication needs to convey the reasons why the values are important; parents who impose values with the rationale of "because I say so" will not usually find their children respecting these dogmatic beliefs. As Ralph Waldo Emerson said, "Who you *are* speaks so loud, I cannot hear what you *say*." The **character** we reveal through **modeling** is the most important influence of all. That is why **parents** are the primary sex educators of their children.

Much has been written about self-acceptance in recent years, including Thomas Harris's *I'm OK, You're OK*. Though it is one of the simplest principles in psychology, it is also one of the most profound. In closing this chapter, we'd like to quote James B. Nelson's thoughts on self-acceptance, from his book *Embodiment*:

> Genuine self-acceptance is basic to humility. Authentic humility is not self-deprecation. It is realistic self-appreciation founded upon the experiential conviction of divine acceptance. It is the security of self that does not compulsively demand narcissistic support and constant affirmation from others. In contrast, self-rejection feeds upon illusions about the self's competence and virtue, often manifesting a need to be universally loved and admired. But such illusions mask a curious combination of arrogance and self-hate, pretense and anger.

CHAPTER THREE

Coming to Terms
with Our Sexuality

A strange alliance of forces in our society has "conspired" to debase the meaning, intent, and value of sex. We know of well-intentioned ministers who claim that if you have sex before marriage, you'll have nothing to look forward to in marriage. If you expect sexual intercourse to be the main goal of marriage, don't marry. It's not worth it. Supersophisticated researchers would have us believe that sex is something you can "quantify," all of which contributes to the disastrous illusion that sex is akin to a gymnastic performance. Some researchers actually want us to take seriously the absurd notion that men reach their sexual peak at age nineteen and women at twenty-nine. Where did they get data like these? A distraught young man once came to us and remarked, "I'm twenty years old and already past my prime, and I haven't even started yet."

Most couples, when asked by researchers about the frequency of their sexual relations, tell an embarrassed lie. The statisticians add up all the lies and come up with an average of 2.2 sexual interludes a week. Why should it matter how many times a week a couple has sexual intercourse? The fact is that there are happily married couples who have sexual relations less than once a month and unhappily married couples who engage in sexual intercourse every day. As far as we can determine, there is no connection between the frequency of sexual intercourse and happiness or mental health. Nor are we impressed with the theorizing of a certain analyst who declared in a recent book that hostility was the "major force in enhancing sexual excitement."

We have often felt that many, if not most, studies in the area of human sexuality are based on a series of false assumptions—carefully documented by research. We may well ask, where is privacy? Where is love? Where is individuality? We are not against research, but we are for the rights of people—especially the right not to compare oneself with anyone else's "norm." We want to put sex into perspective. We see sexual intercourse as one aspect of a relationship; it is important, but not overwhelmingly so. In fact, sexual intercourse is, at best, number nine on our list of the ten most important characteristics of a mature marriage:

1. Love, sensitivity, and respect for each other and a sense of lifetime commitment.
2. Honest communication and support for full self-expression.
3. The freedom to have private thoughts and experiences.
4. A conscious sense of the essential equality of the relationship.
5. A sense of humor—even about occasional failures.
6. Playfulness (physical and verbal), which includes affectionate displays.
7. Respect for "Don't feel like it."
8. Ability to enjoy foreplay and "afterglow."
9. Sexual intercourse.
10. Sharing responsibilities, including household tasks.

Occasionally, when we present this list to an audience, an outraged male suggests that we are talking nonsense—how could sex be number nine? Our reply is, "Because there are eight things more important. And, besides, of the 3,243 really important aspects of a relationship, sex is one of the top ten. Not bad."

It didn't surprise us when Shere Hite (in *The Hite Report*) found that most women she interviewed enjoyed hugging, kissing, cuddling, closeness, and conversations as much as sexual intercourse. Overall, intimacy was more important than orgasms.

It is understandable and no cause for embarrassment that many parents are threatened by certain topics; few people reach adulthood without some areas of inhibition or difficulty. Parents do well to examine these areas realistically. The feeling of being uncomfortable may not disappear. If parents are able to acknowledge their discomfort when discussing a sensitive subject with a child, they can help the child deal with his or her own feelings. Otherwise, children sense by the parent's words or mood that this is an area filled with anxiety and guilt, and that it is better not to discuss it.

Acknowledging an occasional vulnerability to one's children also casts the parent in a more realistic light. For example, "I made a mistake when I insisted that you do the dishes a certain way—I don't even do them that way myself! Sorry to be so bossy—I'm sure you can figure it out for yourself." Or, "I've been reading and thinking about some new ways of working things out in our family...." The aura of perfection that the parent may try to maintain can place impossible demands on the child, who realizes that he or she can't be perfect. Thus, nothing the child does is ever good enough, and self-esteem sinks even further.

It is in this context that we shall now elaborate on some crucial aspects of sexuality—as an aid in helping you explore and evaluate your own sexual behavior, knowledge, and feelings. This represents our judgment based on forty years of study, research, counseling, and teaching. We add to that our bias for common sense and respect for individual differences in preference to what is called "hard data." We present here twenty concepts, in no particular order.

1. *Normal and abnormal.* Normal sexual behavior **among adults** is defined by its being voluntary, nonexploitive, nonabusive, and consensual. In normal relationships, the partners check with each other and imagine how the other is feeling. They are concerned with the safety, health, and well-being of the partner. Normal couples experiment and explore what works best for both of them. Generally, this behavior not only is pleasurable and guilt-free but also enhances self-esteem.

It's easy to classify behavior as abnormal when it doesn't conform to what you know. Sexual behavior is abnormal only when it is compulsive (involuntary), exploitive, abusive, nonconsensual, or guilt-ridden. It generally lowers self-esteem. More often than not it is a "defense" against feelings of depression or inferiority of which the person may not even be aware. Sometimes it is an act of violence, as in the case of rape. If you feel any of these things are happening in your own or your child's relationships, it's time to change!

2. *Sexual preference.* No sensible person need worry that heterosexuality as a primary lifestyle will disappear. The **real** concern in today's world is overpopulation—not sexual preference. (After all, it took millions of years—until 1830—to reach one billion people on Earth and only one more century to reach two billion, in 1930; sixty years later—1990—we had five billion, and today it's almost six billion, with another billion due in fourteen years! Even in America there were one million neglected or abused children in need of adoption in 1997.)

A person's basic sexual orientation is probably determined by the age of five years. This is the position of most respected scholars in the field. Yet it also seems evident that some people's sexuality is not rigidly fixed. Some go through stages of sexual preference at different times of their lives.

3. *All thoughts are normal.* Sexual thoughts, wishes, dreams, and daydreams are normal. No matter how "far out," they cannot, in themselves, hurt you. **Guilt is the energy for the repetition of fantasies that are unacceptable to you.**

Almost everyone with some degree of imagination has, from time to time, fantasies of murder, sadism, incest, or rape. And that's where they stay—just fantasies. As a matter of fact, accepting one's "unacceptable" thoughts as normal is the best way of keeping them under voluntary control. People who constantly repress their fantasies or become preoccupied with them because of guilt are the ones most likely to be harmful to themselves or others.

Here are two examples. A man walks down the street and notices a woman who captures his fancy. He thinks about having an affair with her. The woman doesn't know about it, his wife doesn't know about it, and he enjoys his walk. The sexual imagery is part of a huge, well-developed repertoire of fantasies.

A fifteen-year-old boy catches a glimpse of his thirteen-year-old sister taking a shower. The first thought that comes into his mind is to have sexual intercourse with her. He feels terribly guilty and cannot free his mind from the image or the sexual wish. Nobody in his family understands why he begins avoiding his friends, becomes hostile to his sister, and gets more and more depressed. The fantasy becomes an involuntary repetition of ideas. After a while he forgets (represses) the incident, and only the hostility to his sister remains. If this fellow only understood that his impulse was normal, it would have remained with him for a brief duration (whether or not it was enjoyable) and nothing would have happened.

There are two kinds of guilt: *mature* and *immature*. Mature guilt is a response to something you did wrong. It helps people organize themselves and allows them to respond more rationally to similar future situations. Mature guilt can help you feel better about yourself. Immature guilt, on the other hand, saps your energy; it disorganizes and overwhelms you. You can usually tell if your guilt is immature if it is an **overreaction**, either to something you did wrong or, more commonly, to something you just thought about. Usually immature guilt is a way of expressing hostility toward yourself and is accompanied by feelings of depression. Almost everyone at some time or other has immature guilt.

Most people have sexual thoughts when they are masturbating, having sexual intercourse, and at other (sometimes less convenient) times. **Almost** all reasonably healthy people **at times** find their fantasies more exciting than reality. As long as the fantasies are not accompanied by guilt, it doesn't matter what they are. Only obsessions are harmful—not fleeting thoughts.

4. *Sexual arousal.* Popular culture, especially the mass media, creates the notion that there are standard stimuli for getting aroused. Men, for example, are supposed to be aroused by the "pretty girl" selling automobiles or by actresses in thong bathing suits advertising *Baywatch.* That's all right—except that men who aren't aroused by current fashions of beauty often feel compelled to fake it. The fact is that human beings are sexually aroused by an endless variety of stimuli! **Not** knowing that **all** forms of arousal are all right is what causes trouble. The problem is somewhat more acute with men only because they can't always hide obvious erections.

Some people feel guilty if they are sexually aroused when playing with children, roughing it with dogs, being attracted to their parents, sitting in moving vehicles, having sadistic fantasies, or looking at erotica. If one can accept the arousal experience without guilt, no harm is done. What if, at times, one partner gets excited only or mainly by thoughts or acts that the other finds unacceptable or exploitive? Then you can talk about it, share your feelings, and listen to responses. (There may be a creative, mutually acceptable solution!)

To most sober people, bans on pornography constitute political weapons that threaten a resurgence of the days when even authors such as James Joyce and D. H. Lawrence were considered obscene. Some people want to ban J. D. Salinger's *Catcher in the Rye* from public and school libraries. Museums have been threatened with withdrawal of support if they don't discontinue allegedly "obscene" exhibits.

We know from literally hundreds of studies that even "hard-core" material designed entirely to appeal to our so-called "base instincts" is usually not harmful. In fact, pornography seems to help some people contain their potentially dangerous sexual impulses, and many teenagers have a natural curiosity about it. Usually it represents a passing phase, but if pornography becomes their main understanding of sex, it can have a harmful effect. With the increasing proliferation of hard-core pornography, it is all the more important that parents provide the opportunities for accurate information and open discussion about sex.

5. *Women's liberation.* Some people have come to associate the women's liberation movement only with issues such as abortion, day care, and assertive behavior, but liberation is much more than this. Liberation means that you are attempting to discover yourself in a realistic rather than a culturally stereotyped manner, and then act on your discoveries. Explaining these new feelings and actions is one of the most important bridges that men and women must build.

6. *Masturbation.* Nearly all professionals these days say that masturbation is all right. Then there is a pause—"It's all right if you don't do it too much." And nearly everyone is asking the question "How much is too much?"

Masturbation is a normal sexual expression for all people, no matter at what age or stage in life they happen to be—child, teenager, young adult, middle-aged, elderly, single, or married.

Masturbation causes no physical harm, no matter how frequently it is performed. Men need not worry that their sperm supply is affected, or that they are expending "energy" necessary for sports or other enterprises. A wet dream (nocturnal emission in males) and orgasm stimulated by dreams in women are as natural as any form of sexual expression.

The idea that people who masturbate "a lot" (what's a lot?) don't make friends or are selfish is just plain silly. Eating, talking, sleeping, and masturbating are examples of "natural" behavior that can be compulsive, and thus symptomatic of problems. This does not make eating, talking, sleeping, and masturbating "unnatural."

Though they seldom admit it, some men and women achieve their best orgasms by masturbating. A lot of married people with satisfactory sex lives also masturbate. Some people masturbate hardly at all or not at all, and that's all right, too. Guilt about masturbation is about the only thing that's not desirable.

7. *Telling the truth about your sexual past.* This may be a good thing, but you should make sure that you are telling the truth for the right reasons. Sometimes people reveal "the past" in order to hurt or express hostility toward their partners. Others want to know the past for ulterior purposes. It is not a sign of love to "let it all hang out." We are entitled to privacy in some aspects of our lives. (We favor honesty about the sexual "present" and about feelings and desires.)

8. *Coitus.* Many myths are perpetuated by "sexperts." There is no special amount of time a man's penis is supposed to stay in a woman's vagina in order to guarantee satisfaction. For some, it's thirty seconds—for others, a couple of minutes. It can vary from time to time. The presumed norm of fifteen minutes is ridiculous; many couples find this amount of time too long. There are no standards for everyone or even almost everyone. Each couple must discover what is most enjoyable for them.

One can have sexual pleasure **without** intercourse, orgasm, or simultaneous or multiple orgasm. The media has created the myth that these things are essential. There are many ways couples can enjoy sex. Mutual pleasuring and/or masturbation are alternatives.

9. *Female orgasms.* More nonsense has been written about this subject than about any other area of sexuality. Women have been made to feel so insecure that some need a *Good Housekeeping Seal* to certify their orgasms. Often they pose the question in a serious way to a professional: "How can I tell if I have an orgasm?" And just as often the professional will respond

with an idiotic answer like "If you had one, you'd know it." This response only reinforces a woman's insecurity.

Orgasm is mainly a psychological phenomenon—with associated physical sensations. We define orgasm as a very brief, intensely pleasurable sensual experience accompanied by a series of genital contractions. Orgasm is not always necessary in order to enjoy sexual intimacy.

Most women who enjoy their own bodies, have good feelings about themselves, and like the idea of sexual intimacy have orgasms:

- If they are not intent on having one each time.
- If their partner doesn't ask each time, "Did you have one?" (What kind of conversation is that, anyway?)
- If they feel comfortable about masturbating.

Male orgasms. The best-kept male secret is the myth that every time a male ejaculates he has an orgasm. This simply is not true. Any man who denies it either is not telling the truth or is unaware. Sometimes a man will ejaculate and feel nothing at all. At times there is a little pleasure and at times a great deal. Orgasms vary in strength and pleasure. We suspect that men sometimes fake orgasms. Male orgasm is just as much a psychological phenomenon as is the female orgasm.

10. *Size of genitals and breasts.*

Penis. An all-American hang-up! Men worry whether theirs is BIG enough. Have any of you males noticed men looking around in public bathrooms or showers to see if they can find one smaller than their own? Freud got it wrong. It's **men** who have penis envy. Size has nothing to do with giving or receiving sexual pleasure. What's more, one cannot tell the size of a penis by looking at it when it is **not erect.**

Vagina. Women needlessly worry that their partner's penis is either too small for satisfaction or too big ("painful") for their "small" vagina. When we recall that the vagina is very stretchable and accommodates the birth of a baby, it is not difficult to appreciate that genital size itself is not a factor in pleasure or pain.

Breasts. Breast size or shape has nothing to do with sexual or personal adequacy. In the early stages of puberty, girls often worry because of uneven or late breast development in comparison to their friends.

Many females with large breasts are as self-conscious as those with small ones. The "styles" swing back and forth. Don't let style mess you up.

11. *Sublimation.* People used to think (and some still do) that one could sublimate sex—i.e., propel it into "higher channels" without direct expression—by being creative, athletic, doing charitable work, or becoming a priest or nun.

Adult sexuality can only be

- Expressed,
- Repressed, or
- Suppressed;

it cannot be sublimated!

Individuals who repress their sexuality have a great potential for problems. Repressed sexuality is often revealed in the following ways:

- Physical disorders
- Immaturity
- Revulsion in response to natural functions of the body
- Meanness
- Obsessive–compulsive disorders
- Fears of homosexuality
- Failure to achieve orgasm
- A few other odds and ends

There are some emotionally mature people who choose to remain celibate. They are usually able to acknowledge, but suppress, impulses toward sexual relations or masturbation.

Many people who are emotionally immature have an active, vigorous sex life, as do many people who are emotionally mature. The range of sexual expression as it relates to maturity is infinite.

12. *Normal sex problems.* Just about everybody sometimes has an unsatisfactory sexual experience—unable to "perform" despite wishing they could. An occasional experience of impotence, premature ejaculation, or lack of sexual desire is not uncommon. If you don't panic, the situation will improve. If you attach too much importance to what would otherwise be a temporary problem, it can get worse.

13. *Role playing (positions and techniques).* Sexual relationships thrive on variety. One or both partners can be either active or passive. Just as one can care for someone or be taken care of, bathe someone or be bathed, massage or be massaged, one can play different roles. No one need be frozen in an assigned role. Traditional concepts of what is supposed to be male and female (or active and passive) no longer apply, if they ever really did.

What counts is communication and intimacy—sexual rapport. Roles, positions, and techniques are only the mechanical how-tos in a loving, responsive relationship.

14. *Sexual desire.* Feeling horny is not mainly physiological, biological, constitutional, or hereditary. It is primarily a psychological phenomenon. If you feel turned on and your spouse has a headache (which is lasting for days), consider masturbating. If you have a mature (not guilt-ridden) attitude toward self-pleasuring, you will feel better afterward.

15. *Homosexuality.* It is no longer believed that homosexuality is caused by any one thing or even by a special combination of factors. Homosexuals exist in every culture and society. Ancient

Greek culture found homosexuality acceptable. Our culture has frowned upon it in the past; now public attitudes are undergoing profound positive change.

Homosexuality[1] is not exclusively hereditary, biological, chemical, or constitutional. We wonder sometimes how homophobia interferes with people's natural impulses. Men in our society can be especially frightened by normal desires for intimacy with other males because of their fear of being considered homosexual.

In any case, we now know that homosexual experiences are not rare during childhood and adolescence. These experiences do not necessarily mean that a person will be gay as an adult. One and even some homosexual experiences don't make a person homosexual, any more than one or some heterosexual experiences make a person heterosexual.

It is a false assumption that a person who has homosexual thoughts or dreams must be a homosexual. Mature people are aware that they have both homosexual and heterosexual feelings, even though most prefer sexual activities with members of the opposite sex. In this connection, it might be helpful to point out that it is not easy to judge a person's sexual orientation by appearance. Some "feminine" looking men or "masculine" looking women are heterosexual, and some macho "all-American" men are homosexual.

People who are afraid of their healthy sexual impulses have a problem, no matter what their sexual orientation.

Sexual orientation does not determine whether a person is mature or "normal." Saying that a person is a homosexual tells us no more about the person than saying that a person is a heterosexual.

People have the right, without stigma or coercion, to be who they are. If some 90 percent of the population are heterosexual, that's their business. If perhaps 10 percent express themselves by homosexual, bisexual, or no overt sexual behavior, that's their

---

1. A composite term for both male and female.

business as well. The government has no right to have any say about sexual relations between two consenting adults.

(We hope that there will come a time when people's private, consensual sexual preferences will be of little or no legislative interest and certainly none of anybody else's business!)

16. *"Perversion."* This is an old-fashioned word often used to describe what some people find revolting. For example, there are people who consider anal or oral sex perverted. The word "perversion" is sometimes used to describe such deviant behavior as exhibitionism, masochism, sadism, fetishism, voyeurism, necrophilia, and bestiality.

We think there is nothing wrong with any kind of sex between adults in private if **each partner is nonexploitive and the act is voluntary.** Anal and oral sex are enjoyable for many people and are also ways to have sexual pleasure for those who don't want to (or can't) have sexual intercourse.[2]

If we use the word "perversion" at all, it should be restricted to sexual behaviors that are harmful to another person. This refers to sexual activity that is usually compulsive and guilt-ridden. Examples might be a male who gets his kicks from displaying his penis in a public place or a woman who enjoys intercourse only when she causes physical pain to her partner.

We all have "perverted" feelings at times. They are neurotic and harmful only when they are translated into behavior, or obsessively repeated.

17. *Fear of other people's preferences.* It's all right to have sexual preferences. It is not necessary to enjoy or "be into" anal, oral, auto, homo-, or group sexuality in order to be "with it." Nevertheless, if you have fixed, powerful emotions of revulsion or

---

2. Because of the current concern with AIDS, this position must be restricted to monogamous partners who are reasonably secure about each other's sexual histories. Nevertheless, heterosexuals may underestimate their risk of contracting AIDS—remember, you may not know the sexual history of your partner.

disgust in response to behavior that is enjoyable to others, counseling may be helpful.

18. *Immature, neurotic, or immoral sex.* Sexual practices can be manifestations of immature or neurotic behavior. Here are four of the more common types:

- Compulsive masturbation. You do it not because you like to, but because you can't help it.
- Compulsive heterosexual or homosexual behavior (even if not forced on the other person). This behavior takes place outside an interest in a relationship. It does not enhance or enrich the person and it rarely provides more than momentary relief. A person who is always "on the make" is rarely capable of a sustained relationship and, despite boasting to the contrary, usually does not enjoy sex.
- Excessive compliance. You can be talked into having sex when you really don't want to; before you feel ready for it; with someone you really don't care about; and without using birth control.
- Fetishism and other compulsions. Your main type of sexual outlet is to transfer your attachments to a thing (shoe, undergarment, dress); or you are compelled to expose yourself, steal, or secretly view others (voyeurism) as a form of sexual expression.

And here are the Seven Deadly Sins of immoral sex:

- Rape, molestation and sexual assault
- Hurting, forcing, deceiving, exploiting, and corrupting
- Sexually irresponsible behavior (such as a man abandoning a woman he has impregnated)
- Perpetuating the double standard (demanding rights that you refuse to give your partner, on the basis of gender)
- Sex stereotyping

- Sexual harassment of women or men
- Lying to young children about the facts of life

19. *First experiences of sexual intercourse.* Many first experiences of sex are not pleasurable, despite stories to the contrary. This is especially true if you are too young, too immature, or on your honeymoon.

It is especially important not to diagnose yourself on the basis of these experiences. Men think they are sexual freaks if they are impotent or ejaculate prematurely on their first encounters. Women feel that they are not sexual or feminine if they don't have an orgasm the first time around.

It is surprising how many people have acknowledged that their first sexual experiences were empty, flat—even repulsive.

20. *On being sexually attractive.* People who are self-accepting are sexually attractive to some other individuals, period. It doesn't matter what the cosmetic and toothpaste industries have to say about it.

It's not that short, fat, or "unattractive" people can't find or hold a mate. Instead, people who hate themselves and express it in being (not looking) unattractive, shortsighted, or fatuous tend to repel rather than attract others.

Using certain perfumes, hair tonics, vaginal sprays, or positions will get you nowhere. **Being kind, empathic, and authentic attracts.**

In later chapters we shall be delving deeper into some of the important concepts presented here. However, we hope that this was a good way to introduce you to our basic orientation and to help you examine your own attitudes about sexuality so that you may become a more askable parent.

CHAPTER FOUR

Becoming an Askable Parent

Although parents are expected to be the primary sexuality educators of their own children, survey after survey reveals that they often fail in the task. Even parents who think they have done a good job would be sadly surprised to hear the opinions of their children: "My parents? You must be kidding!" "I learned a little from my friends, only to find out after I left home that most of what I thought I knew was not true."

Let's try to put to rest two myths that are partly responsible for the ever-increasing incidence of irresponsible sexual behavior among the young.

The first myth is that today's young people already know everything there is to know about sex. Some do, of course, but research reveals a staggering ignorance about critical issues. A Johns Hopkins University study of adolescent girls found that 59 percent did not know when in the menstrual cycle the risk of conception was greatest. Worse, young people with little sexual experience will often feel compelled to exaggerate the extent of their activities.

Don't believe the stories that young people knowingly take risks, or that girls from disadvantaged homes deliberately try to get pregnant. Research on teenage pregnancy usually involves asking pregnant girls if they had originally wanted to conceive. In one such study of three hundred teenagers (in a single high school), we asked why the girls hadn't practiced birth control.

"Oh, but we did," was the general response.
"I used one of my mother's pills."
"I didn't think I could get pregnant standing up."
"He said he'd pull out in time."
"I didn't think I could get pregnant the first time."

When we asked three hundred sexually active but not yet pregnant girls if they wanted to get pregnant, a full 90 percent said they did not. A typical comment was, "Do you think I'm stupid? I'm only fourteen." Furthermore, in surveys of high school students, more than 90 percent did not know that the original symptoms of venereal disease disappear after a while. Most assumed that the disappearance of the symptoms meant that the disease had been cured. A majority of the same students did not know that females generally have no symptoms at all when they are infected with gonorrhea or chlamydia.

Some readers may already be thinking that their own children are not involved in sexual experimentation. It should be remembered that, whether anyone likes it or not (including the teenagers themselves), more than 70 percent of all high-school students will have had sexual intercourse before graduation.

Each year we received hundreds of poignant letters from teenagers. A number begin something like this: "I'm fifteen, pregnant, and I can't tell my folks (they'll kill me). What should I do?" More typical are those such as this one:

I come from a family where I have learned sex from my friends. My mother don't mention it to me. And I still don't know what most of sex and love is all about. So I would like to know because I'm only 14 years of age. And I've seen my friends get pregnant. I'd like to know what it's all about. Thank you.

The 1.3 million teenage pregnancies in the United States in 1998 and the millions of new cases of sexually transmitted diseases (STDs) among persons under 25 belie the myth that young people "know it all."

The second myth is that knowledge is harmful. Virtually all opposition of sex education is based on the assumption that children who "know about sex" will practice it. Even editors of metropolitan newspapers often blame sex education for the rise of illegitimate births and venereal disease. Yet, as we will detail later, for the vast majority of American students, sex education is simply absent from the curriculum.

Our research tells us that young people who do not understand "the facts of life" are more likely to make mistakes. In fact, well-informed young people are more likely to delay sexual experiences, at least until after they finish high school, and then to use effective contraception.

THE PARENT'S ROLE

Most parents, after all, want to educate their children about sexuality. They realize that schools, churches, community organizations, and the mass media (including rock music and ads with false information and confusing innuendo) can offer only bits and pieces and cannot be expected to reflect their personal values. Many parents also fear that too much information too soon will overstimulate their children—will arouse otherwise dormant sex impulses. This attitude is the first of many roadblocks to effective sex education in the home.

Unlike a few experts in this field, we've never been able to discover a documented case of a child's having been overstimulated by facts alone. Should parents err by offering too much information, children will simply get bored, turn them off, or cut the conversation short with an unrelated question. Fear, unresolved curiosity, and ignorance are far more likely to result in overstimulation than are facts, lovingly offered. Our campaign against ignorance has led some opponents of sex education to tell jokes about us. A popular example: A child asks where she came from, and her mother responds with an elaborate explanation of the seed and the egg. At the end, the amazed child explains that she only wanted to know if she came from Philadelphia. To this, our response is a giggle and a simple retort: "So what? Now the child knows not only where she was born, but *how* she was born."

Quite understandably, many parents who did not receive sex education in their own homes feel uncomfortable talking about sexuality with their children. There is no instant remedy for such feelings, but it may be helpful to ask the question: Who is really comfortable about anything these days? Contrary to modern theory, it simply is not necessary to feel entirely comfortable about sexuality in order to communicate effectively with your children.

As the primary force in your child's life, you are providing sexuality education in one form or another no matter what you do. The question is not *whether* you will teach your children about sex—that question has been settled! What remains is *how well*. Silence teaches no less eloquently than speech. If you convey to a young child, or a teenager, the impression that you feel a bit awkward discussing love and sex, chances are good that you'll score. Your child might well respond to your honesty with affection and appreciation, with a hug and a kiss and verbal reassurances that your discomfort is perfectly understood. Many an anxious parent has been happily surprised to hear a child say, "Don't worry, Mom! It's all right."

Parents who worry that they don't know enough about the subject to be effective teachers ought to pause and consider this question: How much is it really necessary to know? To a particularly technical or baffling question, a parent can always respond with the truth: "I don't know, but I'll look it up for you and tell you tomorrow." "Let's look it up together" would be an even better response. A small child's questions can usually be answered with a few words of elementary explanation. Older children are more likely to ask questions about values than about anatomy. Even so, with excellent books no more distant than your local library, what excuse do you really have for remaining silent?

Sometimes parents conceive of children growing up in "stages"—be they fashioned by Gesell, Freud, Kohlberg, Erikson, or Piaget. Frankly, as interesting and as creative as these theories are, we rarely see real children progress in an orderly sequence. Children are full of surprises. Concepts that some intelligent children understand at three and four still baffle others at nine and ten (even when the measured IQs are similar). Peer groups differ in the words they use, and some children are more comfortable and more ready for more specific language at an earlier age (e.g., vagina, penis, urination), though words are never as important as attitudes.

We are interested in this phenomenon because we often hear warnings about not giving children sexual information before their "stage" has arrived. We encourage parents not to worry about offering information before a child can wholly comprehend it. Haven't you noticed that complicated fairy tales are fascinating to children whether they understand them all or not? They'll simply get what they can, and the rest goes over their head. Either way, it's OK.

Use common sense, but respond to all questions regardless of stage. Remember that children at different ages will often ask what you believe are questions already answered. "Where did I come from?" asked at age five is not the same question when posed at nine or ten. Some children will never ask questions regardless of the stage they're supposed to be in, and some will begin to ask highly abstract questions before they are supposed to be able to do so. Parents are far less likely to go "wrong" by responding to children's questions with perhaps a little more information than they believe the child can handle, than they are by underestimating the child's capabilities.

Some parents are concerned about making honest mistakes or giving wrong answers. Parents should realize that they can make mistakes without harming their children. The following examples may be illustrative.

A child wanders into the bedroom while you and your spouse are having sexual intercourse. You tell the child, "Leave," then worry that you have been too harsh. In the morning you can apologize for not having said, "Please leave." Then you can explain what you were doing. If your child asks to watch the next time, kindly but firmly explain that sex is private. A child may not understand the prohibition, but later in life he or she will grow to appreciate the concept of privacy. Most important, learn to laugh at the outrageous proposition that a child who has witnessed sexual intercourse will need years of analysis to get over it. The person who, as a child, never once saw his or her parents being naturally and openly affectionate is a more likely candidate for analysis.

Perhaps you are worried about your neighbors' response if your child were to tell the truth about sex to some friends. Their parents hear about it and inform you, in no uncertain terms, of their horror and indignation. We don't think you should be swayed by their attitudes. Your responsibility is to tell your children the truth without instructions to keep it confidential. If your neighbors don't like it, that's their problem. And remember, no matter what parents do, children will share whatever information they have about sex; it's about time that well-educated children become an important neighborhood resource with respect to sex education. We realize that your child may be deprived of a playmate, but in the long run this kind of sensitive experience could contribute to your child's being more creative, happier, and better adjusted.

NINETEEN KEY QUESTIONS

Of the thousands of questions we get from parents, the following are the most common. It is not expected that you will agree with all our responses, which express our personal bias.

1. When should I tell?

The answer is simple: It is time to tell whenever the child asks. If you are an **askable** parent, your children may come to you with questions about sex from the time they are two or three years old. Young children's questions are sometimes nonverbal. For example, a child may constantly follow you into the bathroom. To encourage them, you could say, "It looks like you're wondering about something—can I guess what it is?"

Some shy children might ask no questions at all, even of the most askable parents. If your child hasn't raised sexuality-oriented questions by age five, you should start the conversation. Read a book with your child. Tell him or her about a neighbor or a relative who is going to have a baby. While it's fine on occasion to make analogies to animals, do not concentrate on them in your explanations. People and animals have very different habits.

2. How much should I tell?

You should tell your child a *bit* more than you feel he or she can understand.

3. How explicit should I be?

Make it a point to use the correct terminology. Avoid such childish expressions as "pee-pee" or "wee-wee." Say directly that when a husband and a wife love each other and want to have a baby, the man puts his penis into the woman's vagina. If the sperm from the man's body joins with the egg (or ovum) inside the woman's body at the right time, a baby gets started. Depending upon the child's age and other factors, you might say more: "Sometimes it takes a year or two before a child gets started." Or, "Your father (or mother) and I enjoy loving each other in this way but right now we're not making a baby because our family isn't ready for another child yet."

The main idea is that parents can be explicit without over-stating the case or feeling compelled to describe sexual relations to a child who hasn't yet grasped much more basic ideas. It is also wiser to say at the start that a baby has its beginning in the mother's uterus, not the stomach, because a child's imagination can easily picture the fetus being mixed up with the food.

4. Is there such a thing as giving too much sex education too soon?
Parents worry a great deal about whether they can "harm" their children with "too much" information or by telling their children things that they won't understand. Let us state again that despite the protests of a few "experts," knowledge is not harmful. It does not matter if the child doesn't understand everything you say. What counts is that you are an askable parent. If the child can trust you not to be rigid or hostile in your response or to give mis-information, he or she will ask you questions and use you as a source of wisdom and guidance. This is more important than ever in an era when children are bombarded by titillation from televi-sion in their living rooms, or even their bedrooms!

5. What about nudity in the home?
Some parents are relaxed about undressing in front of young children or bathing with them and some aren't, but there will always be times when it happens. These are good opportunities for children to ask important questions: "How come you have one and I don't?" "How come yours is bigger than mine?" "How come you have two and I don't have any?" "How come you're fancy and I'm plain?" Parents should respond directly to these and similar questions.

A question also arises when a child wants to touch a parent's genitals or breasts. There are several acceptable responses, one of which is simply that you don't want him or her to do this. Even if children protest against that familiar double standard—"But *you* touch *me*"—you can explain that this is because you have to bathe them and keep them clean. In any case, don't make a big thing out of it. A child's own growing sense of modesty will tell you when to start undressing in private. When a child wants to go to the bathroom alone or to undress without an audience, parents need to respect that developing sense of privacy.

6. Is too much masturbation harmful?

Masturbation is a normal expression of sexuality at any age. Once this is clear to the child, he or she will not feel guilty and thus will be much less likely to become a compulsive masturbator. It is guilt that creates the energy for compulsive masturbation. That masturbation is a private activity needs to be made clear, and all children old enough to understand the concept of privacy can be taught this. (Mary Calderone, when asked at a lecture how she got interested in the field of sex education, answered, "Because I had to wear gloves until I was eight years old." At that time, it was thought that making a child wear gloves would inhibit them from masturbating.)

7. What about the use of obscenities?

Children use vulgar language to find out what it means, to get a rise out of their parents, or to test a new and powerful weapon. If a child uses an obscenity, the parent should quickly and calmly explain its meaning, perhaps using the word itself in the explanation. Even the most common four-letter word can be handled in this way, provided the parent explains its gross intent as well as the fact that it's a crude synonym for sexual intercourse. There is an advantage in using the obscenity itself in your explanation and modeling relaxed and understanding attitudes. Thereafter the word can hardly be used by the child as a "weapon."

8. What about the child who likes to look at his father's Playboy magazines or at the nude photographs that are becoming more common in ordinary magazines?
There is no harm in this. In fact, it may provide an opportunity for teachable moments. You might point out that not all people look like that and state simply that men sometimes like to look at nude photographs of women and women sometimes enjoy looking at photographs of nude men. No big deal.

Hard-core pornography is something else again. Though it has not been proved harmful, it is clearly not educational, and parents would understandably prefer to keep their children away from it. Although it may not always be possible to shield a child from graphic material (e.g., on the Internet), parents can take some comfort in the fact that people who have received enlightened sexuality education tend to grow bored with pornography quickly.

9. What about embarrassing questions in public?
Children have a great knack for asking the most delicate questions in the supermarket or when special guests have come to dinner. The best approach, no matter how embarrassed you are, is to tell the child that he or she has asked a very good question; if you still have your wits about you, proceed to answer it then and there. In most cases, your guests will silently applaud. If you feel you can't answer the question right away, it is very important to praise the child for asking and to state specifically when you will discuss it. In general, it is better to risk shocking a few grown-ups than to scold or put off your own child.

10. What should I do if my husband thinks it's my job to tell our child about sex?
Sexuality education is properly the responsibility of both parents. It is reflected in their behavior with each other and in communication with children. If your husband refuses to have any part of it, you must take it upon yourself to explain sex and love to all the

children in your family. Incidentally, it has never been established that girls are better educated by their mothers or boys by their fathers. (Single parents, relax.)

11. What can I do to prevent my child from becoming a homosexual?
Some parents have rather strong notions of what constitutes "protection." Contrary to the opinion of some professionals, our view is that there's nothing parents can do to prevent their children from becoming homosexual. No specific attitudes or behaviors have been found to discourage the development of a homosexual orientation. Similarly, there is no convincing evidence that parents can cause homosexuality in their children. It is important to understand that good mental health is not necessarily a function of sexual orientation. Just as homosexual adults can be happy and creative individuals, heterosexual adults can turn to drugs or crime and generally lead unhappy lives.

There are fathers who are reluctant to be affectionate with their sons after age five or six for fear that the child will become homosexual. This is unjustified and very distressing to the child. Some parents overreact to their children's play when it does not conform to long-standing stereotypes—for example, when boys play dress-up in women's clothing or play with dolls, or when girls play tough and like sports. Certain parents are even upset because their young sons like to read a lot! These are rarely signs that the child is growing up homosexual.

Parents should convey an attitude of acceptance for people who have different sexual orientations. With *Ellen* "coming out" and homosexuals still being harassed, we are provided with ample opportunities to discuss this topic.

12. What if my children think I'm old-fashioned?
They will probably be right! Most parents are old-fashioned. Acknowledge it and continue expressing your views without worrying which label your child might attach to them.

13. How can I talk to my teenage daughter about birth control without giving her the message that it's all right for her to have sexual intercourse?
Some parents believe that teenagers equate information with consent. Your teenage children know very well what your values are. It's one thing to tell a daughter that you will disown her if she becomes pregnant; it's quite another to explain your feelings something like this: "We really think you're too young to have sexual intercourse, but if you're not going to listen to us, we urge you to practice birth control. Above all, we don't ever want you to feel that there's anything you can't talk to us about." Starting younger makes it easier, but you can still do it now. Of course this applies to alcohol and other drugs, smoking, and all the issues that cause the hazards of adolescence. The schools feel much more comfortable these days about being proactive on these topics, from a very early age; however, most parents still have to fill the sex education gap.

14. I worry about my children being molested. How can I talk about this without frightening them?
A little-known fact is that as many as 80 percent of all child molestation cases involve someone the child knows, such as a father, a stepparent, or a baby-sitter. About 90 percent of all cases involve a heterosexual male molesting a young child. As part of a family's general discussions about sexuality, children should be taught not to go off with strangers and not to allow anyone to touch their genitals. This is also a good opportunity to teach children about their public and private parts and public and private places. Children can be told that it's not right for anyone to touch their genitals, or for anyone else to ask them to touch theirs, no matter who it is. Here again, there are plenty of instances that will come up on television to precipitate a "talk." Some individuals force children to submit to sexual activities and make them promise never to tell anyone what happened. Should you suspect that your child has been abused in this way, it is essential to make

him or her understand that such promises should not be kept. The fact that most people are decent and kind must be balanced with the reality that some people take advantage of children. A critical point is to discourage a child who has been molested from feeling any guilt or blame whatsoever. Such crimes are always and entirely the responsibility of the adults who committed them. (See our book *Better Safe Than Sorry,* Prometheus Books.)

15. We've never talked about sex. I would like to approach the subject now, but my teenage son absolutely refuses. What should I do?

This is a common situation, and it is appropriate for the parent to begin the conversation something like this: "I really made a mistake by waiting this long and I wish we had talked when you were younger. I can understand why you might feel embarrassed to talk with me." Plan ahead for such discussions; have a book ready. Tell your son that you think he might be interested in it. Explain that some of the material might embarrass him but that you're going to leave the book around just the same. The main thing is for him to understand that you are available to talk anytime he is ready. Another technique is to "hide" a book.[1] Most teenagers are very adept at finding such "hidden" material. Sometimes the best approach is to talk about the subject in general. For example, talk about a sex-related news item in today's newspaper.

Here are some of the most frequently asked questions teenagers report they are **not likely** to ask their parents:

- Am I masturbating too much?
- Do I have homosexual tendencies?
- Am I abnormal if I have thoughts about sex with people I know, even family members?
- Are my breasts too small?

---

1. A fun book to "hide" is *The Teenage Survival Book.* (See Recommended Books.)

- Is my penis too small?
- How can you tell if you have VD?
- Is there something wrong with me if I remain a virgin?
- How can I say no?
- How can I tell if I'm pregnant?
- How come I have all these unexplained erections?

Think back to the time when you were growing up and remember the kinds of questions you had about sexuality. Then you'll be able to better appreciate your child's concerns. (For our suggestions on several of the above questions, refer to the previous chapter.)

16. What if I find my child undressed and playing doctor with a neighbor's child?

This is a fairly common game children play. It must be considered a normal developmental episode for preschool children. The most important thing is for parents not to lose their cool. Convey the message that you understand why they want to play with each other; tell them you'd rather they wouldn't. Indicate that you consider their genitals to be private. Then ask them to get dressed and play other games. It is not appropriate to send the other child home or to make a scene in any way.

17. What is your opinion of high-school students having sexual intercourse?

We're opposed to teenagers having sexual intercourse. They tend to be impulsive, without considering the consequences. The double standard (OK for boys—taboo for girls) is still very much with us. Also, teenage pregnancy is definitely unsound from medical, moral, and psychological points of view. Another reason for this position is that young people for the most part have difficulty using good judgment because of their immaturity, ignorance, and inexperience.

Although we say no to sex for teenagers, no teenager has ever asked for our consent. It is unrealistic for parents to assume that their teenagers will not have sexual relationships in the absence of parental permission. Parents still can exert a **positive** influence. Without anger, you can explain the reasons for waiting. Even young adults who are working or in college could receive similar parental messages. You might acknowledge that the decision is theirs, but if they should choose to engage in sexual intercourse it is their duty, to themselves and to their partners, to act responsibly and use contraception (particularly condoms).

18. What should be the role of public schools in sexuality education?

Sexuality education should be part of the regular curriculum. In most schools, it is currently excluded because of extremist pressures on school boards and administrators (Chapter 5 covers this subject in depth).

19. How can I bring up my children to respect my values?

An excellent question! You are lucky: you happen to be the one person your children will "take after"! Their set of values depends largely on your lifestyle and the kinds of values you exemplify. You as a parent are a model for your children (which, of course, does not imply perfection), and as such you have the best opportunity of anyone they know to foster a true respect for individual differences.

Askable parents feel positive about themselves and communicate well with each other. They also have a sense of humor and recognize that not every untoward event is a trauma. Their children tend to confide in them, recognizing that their parents have a lot of common sense. Askable parents can admit, "I've made a mistake—I don't know everything." Askable parents have a better chance of bringing up children who respect their values than do those who are not responsive to their children's sexual needs and curiosity.

Sexuality Education in the Schools

O ur society devotes much time and energy coping with unwanted pregnancy, sexually transmitted diseases, and related problems (including overpopulation) once they have occurred, and almost none on how to help people prevent them in the first place. As a national effort, sex education[1] has not even been tried. The Welfare Reform Act of 1997 has hampered these efforts even further, by providing funding only for "abstinence-based" programs. The most optimistic estimates suggest that scarcely 10 percent of our nation's young people receive adequate sex education in public schools. The remaining 90 percent are exposed to "sanitized," fragmentary, isolated lectures on basic reproductive facts—the "plumbing" of human sexuality. Since only about 25 percent of parents sex-educate their children, our society persists in producing sexually ignorant, sexually vulnerable citizens.

One apparent paradox is that Gallup and other national pollsters consistently report that between 80 and 85 percent of

---

1. Because of common usage, "sexuality education" and "sex education" will be used interchangeably to mean sexuality education as previously defined.

American adults support sex education in the schools. There were few differences of opinion on this subject between the generations and between geographic locations. The latest Gallup poll results include the following:

- 92 percent support inclusion of information on STDs
- 92 percent support inclusion of information on AIDS
- 89 percent support the inclusion of information on teen pregnancy
- 87 percent support inclusion of information on birth control
- 65 percent support inclusion of information on homosexuality

Every single figure is an increase from 1987 polls.

Do we have proof that sexuality education works? In one sense, this is an unfair question, because there are so few places that have effective programs. In fact, we are not familiar with a single public school system in the entire United States that has a substantive K–12 sex education curriculum.

The National PTA recently did a survey on comprehensive school health programs that shows that the majority of schools either lack or have inadequate comprehensive health programs— especially in the area of mental health. Only 8 to 21 percent of the respondents' schools offered any type of mental health services, with suicide prevention offered least often.

Early research has detailed the benefits of good sex education programs in such places as St. Paul, Minnesota, and Falls Church, Virginia. When we get right down to it, it is extremely difficult to isolate the effects of such programs (just as it would be difficult to conduct research on how civics classes improve citizenship) in the face of such influences as peer group pressure and the commercialization of sex in the media. In any case, the best research now available comes from the work of Professors Zelnik and Kim of Johns Hopkins University. They conclude that young women who have had sex education appear less likely to become pregnant.

Their studies are flawed by the fact that they didn't obtain data on the quality of the sex education received. However, their evidence does suggest that there is not a significant association between taking a course in sex education and being sexually active. In other words, their studies revealed that although sex education does not reduce sexual activity, it does not increase it, either (as some critics maintain).

We favor sex education for its intrinsic healing contribution to the welfare of young people. Simply put: Knowledge in such a crucial personal/social area is worthwhile. It adds up to self-worth, independence, and health in the emerging adult. Our clinical observations over the past forty years suggest something else of great interest. High-school students who are sexually active (engaging in sexual intercourse) are less likely to go to college than those who are virgins (both male and female). The virgins are generally more likely to take leadership roles, have a more active social life, talk more freely with their parents, be in better physical shape, and control rash impulses than are nonvirgins. The virgins are better at postponing immediate gratification in exchange for later success. We can't prove it, but we're willing to wager that most conservatively minded parents have made similar observations.

It is no accident that sex education in the schools is supported by virtually all relevant national professional and parent groups, including these:

- American Academy of Pediatrics
- American Association of School Administrators
- American Federation of Teachers
- American Home Economics Association
- American Library Association
- American Medical Association
- American Psychiatric Association
- American Public Health Association
- American School Health Association

- Girls Clubs of America
- Girls Incorporated
- Latina Roundtable on Health and Reproductive Rights
- National Association of State Boards of Education
- National Education Association Health Information Network
- National School Boards Association
- National Urban League
- United States Conference of Mayors
- Young Women's Christian Association

SIECUS (the Sex Information and Education Council of the United States), a conservative group much vilified by staunch opponents of sex education, has taken the following position on sex education in the schools:

...programs conducted by specially trained educators add an important dimension to the sexuality education given children by their families and religious and community groups. Such programs must be carefully formulated by each community in order to respect the diversity of values and beliefs represented in a public school classroom...with curricula and resources appropriate to the ages of the students.

Yet we are faced with the Great American Hang-up, a secret belief that **knowledge is harmful**—"If you tell kids about sex, they'll do it!" (Of course, they are doing it, but without the benefit of knowledge.) It is self-defeating to continue this myth, especially in light of the barrage of sexual material thrown at them around the clock.

Other questions logically arise: What should be taught? How and by whom should it be taught? Whose values should be conveyed? Sexuality programs cannot be taught without values. While teaching contraception, for example, the instructor must convey some basic values: (a) it is better for psychological and physiological reasons that teenagers not get pregnant, and (b) it is wrong to exploit or hurt other human beings. All other subjects, such as history, social studies, and economics, are taught within the context of value systems. Why should sexuality be an exception?

There is, in teaching, a vast difference between being moral and being moralistic. Moralistic presentations seek to impose a personal point of view in a dogmatic way. It is acceptable to state, for example, that virtually all established religious groups believe it is better to wait until marriage to have sexual intercourse, but it would be moralistic to suggest that if you do engage in sex before marriage, you'll go to Hell. Programs are best taught with a moral perspective that encourages democratic ideals while preserving individual liberty. (See Chapter 6.)

Moral education encourages people to strive toward the accepted ideals of a society and presents facts to facilitate responsible decision-making. This is an important part of any sexuality education curriculum.

Even the most controversial topics may be discussed in school. Subjects such as masturbation, homosexuality, and abortion could be studied in terms of the range of opinions and research that exists. Ways to prevent STD and teenage pregnancy need to be presented. Since there is no denying that people make mistakes (even the president!), alternatives should be presented to teenagers who face these problems. Who, for example, would dispute the need for good prepartum care or for the immediate treatment of oneself and one's partner once a diagnosis of STD is made?

In terms of actual curriculum guidelines, the Virginia Department of Health and Education in 1978 developed the following goals of family-life education. It should help the student to do the following:

• Develop appreciation of the roles played by family members and recognize the ways in which these roles change and interact with one another

- Understand the interpersonal attitudes, skills, and responsibilities that strengthen effective family life
- Develop a positive self-concept
- Grow in understanding of self and others
- Understand their physical and emotional growth and development
- Understand how reproduction occurs and life begins—plant, animal, human
- Understand that heredity and environment influence growth and development
- Understand and develop a wholesome attitude toward human sexuality as a basic factor throughout life
- Build and develop insights and values regarding human sexuality
- Prepare a suitable foundation for responsible adulthood

Clearly, sex education is a responsibility that optimally should be shared by parents, churches, schools, and various government agencies. Toward this end, there are a number of important points to keep in mind, and a number of advocacy roles that would further the cause of producing educated, sexually responsible adults.

Parents can help themselves and their children by enrolling in or organizing adult sex education courses and seminars. They can seek direction from a variety of sources already established in most communities, such as church groups and PTAs. On hundreds of college campuses, at health centers and social agencies, there are sex education workshops organized specifically for teachers, parents, and expectant parents.

It is of the greatest importance that parents support well-planned sex education programs in their children's schools. Parents can attend school board meetings and voice their support for the programs, as well as contribute their ideas on how they should be structured. Write letters to superintendents and principals asking them to incorporate sexuality education curricula into the schools. If a controversy develops over the programs in the local media, don't be afraid to compose a letter to the editor. It is well known that educators are loath to plan and implement sex education when they are unaware of the sentiments of the community; they need and appreciate such input from parents. Parents can work together to develop "immunization education" against predatory ads and TV shows that exploit teens sexually; they can also organize letter-writing campaigns to networks and shows (both those they like and those they don't).

As for teachers, an unflappable demeanor, a strong credibility, a sense of humor, and a compassionate nature are characteristics that are paramount. This is true for all teachers, and especially for those involved in sex education programs. Teachers should be able to establish a genuine rapport with their students and be prepared to help when a student approaches them with a personal problem. Assistance could include referring students to public or private agencies where, for instance, they can obtain confidential tests for pregnancy and STDs, plus follow-up treatment if needed. Some students are reluctant to discuss personal problems or feelings with a school nurse or with their parents, yet many have been known to confide in a teacher they trust. (Teachers can be "askable," too.)

The sensitivity of the subject and the inexperience of school administrators in dealing with a few vocal opponents have contributed to the failure of sex education in the public schools. Nevertheless, many school courses could be enhanced greatly by incorporating information about human sexuality into them. Subjects such as psychology, home economics, English, social studies, and biology lend themselves logically to the inclusion of sex education. Home economics is especially adaptable in this regard, because it is the type of course where the principles of parenting are taught. (Don't assume that this instruction is for girls only; home economics should be mandatory for both sexes.) And there's no reason why topics such as the changing size of the

American family and shifting attitudes toward human reproduction cannot be dovetailed into American and World History courses.

Our view is that a quality sex education program—perhaps more appropriately entitled "Family-Life Education"—must include the following principles:

1. *Enhancing the self-concept*—a prerequisite for establishing mature relationships and acting sexually responsible.
2. *Preparing for marriage and parenthood*—understanding the interpersonal skills and responsibilities that strengthen family life and encouraging lifelong love and commitment.
3. *Understanding love* as the basic component of a person's sexuality, including help in deciding "how you can tell if you are really in love."
4. *Preparing to make responsible decisions* in critical areas of sexuality, based on a universal value of not hurting or using others.
5. *Helping people understand the need for equal opportunities* for males and females. Schools have a responsibility to discourage sexism.
6. *Helping people develop tolerance and appreciation* for people who don't conform to the traditional norms regarding marriage and childbearing.
7. *Contributing to knowledge and understanding of the sexual dimension of our lives*—including the realization that we are sexual beings even *before* birth and have sexual needs and a sexual identity throughout life. It includes an appreciation for the wide range of sexuality; that sexual expression is not limited to heterosexual, genital intercourse; and that sexual expression goes beyond reproduction.

In family-life education, feelings, communication, and values should be the focus. The most successful programs will be those that raise young people's level of self-esteem and teach them the facts of physiology and contraception they need to know. Girls especially must be helped to cope with the double standard, which implies that while boys may experiment sexually, girls may not, or that girls must bear the full responsibility for any offspring resulting from out-of-wedlock births. Young people also need guidance on subtler issues, such as how to respond to the lines that boys in every society use to persuade girls to have sexual relations with them (and vice versa). We can educate them about the lines that are used by ads and jingles to encourage boys to score and girls to be sexual sirens. It takes strength to counteract the sarcasm and cynicism and put-downs of TV comedy as well. Girls can be told that sex is never a test of love, and boys that using another human being to satisfy selfish desires is wrong.

Young people who feel good about themselves and who feel comfortable with their values are more likely to receive information openly and use it to their own best advantage. In this atmosphere, the transmission of values and information through sex education programs is most likely to be successful.

We must make it clear what the extremist opposition is all about. Sexuality education used to be equated with Communism, but that's not very popular anymore. Now the attacks focus on humanism. The American Humanist Association covers a wide range of beliefs that are ethics-based and include theistic as well as nontheistic adherents. (There are similar groups such as the Society for Ethical Culture.) However, people such as Dr. Tim LeHaye claim that *secular humanism* dominates and controls our public-school system. We publicly offered a $10,000 reward if he or anyone could certify that a single public-school system in the entire United States has a secular-humanist curriculum. Dr. LeHaye made inquiries about the reward but has not claimed it. The secular humanists are, in fact, a small group of a few thousand intellectuals who believe that the hatred and divisiveness of religion are now a major threat to global security. Despite their small numbers and

minimal influence, secular humanists have been erroneously identified as the major corrupters of today's youth.

Censorship represents another form of opposition to sex education and is a major problem now in many parts of the country.
The American Library Association's Office of Intellectual
Freedom reports that the number of complaints concerning
books in school and public libraries has increased *tenfold* during
the past decade. The Gablers of Longview, Texas, wanted to ban
from our public schools textbooks that do not agree with their
highly puritanical, idiosyncratic view of what sexuality or patriotism is all about. They were, unfortunately, quite successful in
their campaign. Their main view: "Too many textbooks leave students to make up their own minds about things."

Another attack is to cite Scandinavia as a center of moral decay.
In fact, the Scandinavian countries have higher standards of living
than we do and have almost eliminated poverty. Hitting children is
against the law in Norway, and literacy rates are quite high in all the
Scandinavian countries. Sweden has had mandatory sex education
for the past thirty years, and the evidence is clear that there has
been a significant decline in unintended pregnancies, venereal diseases, and sex crimes there. We thoroughly researched this issue
ourselves while in Sweden and Denmark. One enormous difference
emerged: more than 80 percent of Scandinavian teenagers use birth
control the first time they have sexual intercourse, in contrast to
about 30 percent in the United States.

It would be instructive to quote from *Guidelines for Sex
Education in the Swedish School System*, developed in 1974 and
still in effect. The following are selections from these guidelines
that teachers in "decadent" Sweden are encouraged to teach:

- The Commission has found that the fundamental values indicate that the following ethical guidelines, among others, should
  be maintained and promoted in the course of teaching:
- A worthwhile aim is to combine sexual life, togetherness, and

respect for the integrity of the other person. *This, in the Commission's opinion, is a central value judgment that should set the tone of sex education as a whole.*

- There apply to sexual relationships the same demands for consideration to others and responsibility for the consequences of action as hold in other fields of life. This means, first and foremost, that no fellow being should be regarded exclusively as a means for the satisfaction of another's interests and needs. In the sexual as in other fields, any form of mental pressure or physical violence constitutes a violation of the other person's integrity.

- Teaching should support a standard that is embraced by the great majority of the Swedish population, namely the rejection of "unfaithfulness." By unfaithfulness should be meant in this context a disloyalty rather than a sexual act in itself.

- Teaching should reject the traditional double morality by which moral sentence is passed upon women for actions that a man can commit with impunity. The rejection of sexual double morality is one aspect of the function of teaching to combat prejudice regarding sexual roles.

- The demand for equal rights entails also that teaching should argue against racial discrimination in the sexual field. As immigration continues, this question can become increasingly topical.

- The condemnation of variations in the direction of people's sexual urge should be counteracted and a considerate attitude to such phenomena promoted.

- Teaching should promote recognition of the right to a sexual life on the part of the physically and mentally handicapped, the mentally diseased, the inmates of prisons, and others tied to institutions. Prejudice against the sexual life of the elderly should be combated.

- Teaching should proclaim sexual tolerance in the sense of respecting the rights of others to speak for and live by sexual standards that one rejects. Such tolerance, however, cannot apply to attitudes in the sexual field which are incompatible with the fundamental values which have to be promoted. Teaching, for instance, cannot take a tolerant view of racial discrimination in this field or of double morality.

Proposals thus far have examined the fundamental values that teaching should maintain and promote. Among the *controversial values* the Commission lists the following, which should thus be treated without taking sides.

Ethical attitudes toward abortion. On this question some groups consider that abortion should only occur on specific medical and other grounds, while others consider that the wishes of the woman should be paramount. The school cannot be involved in arguments in favor of either point of view. It is of the greatest importance, however, that the arguments of both groups be correctly reported. (This has become a crucial issue here as fewer and fewer doctors are willing to perform abortions because of the violence practiced by antiabortionists, e.g., bombing clinics and harassing and murdering doctors.)

Premarital sexual relationships with the person one intends to marry or permanently live with are regarded as self-evidently acceptable by the great majority of the Swedish population. About half of those with a personal Christian faith, however, are convinced that sexual life together in accordance with God's will can take place only within marriage. Such parents and their children must be able to assume that their view will be presented in the schools in a proper and respectful manner. Teaching must not take sides against their view. It is another matter that teaching must devote considerable time to the questions of personal premarital relationships. The results? In 1999 teen pregnancies are uncommon, and there are few cases of HIV/AIDS. Sexuality educators in Sweden accept the view that the great majority of Swedish youths are responsible!

We can learn a lot from the Swedes! There are parents who love and want the best for their children and who are also uncertain about sexuality education in the schools. We encourage such parents to become involved in the planning and implementation of sex education programs so that they can see for themselves what is going on. In fact, school-based programs need the commitment of more concerned parents who share a vital interest in their children's welfare.

We believe that once parents who oppose sexuality education understand the programs better, they will choose to support them.

The bulk of the opposition to sex education comes from small, articulate, well-organized extremist and sometimes fanatical groups. If they represent 5 percent of the population, we would be astonished. Nevertheless, superintendents and principals of schools are invariably overly responsive to these groups. They want to avoid controversy. Some administrators and school boards have lost sight of the fact that wrestling with controversial issues is at the very heart of the democratic process.

Interestingly enough, school systems that do have programs—such as the state of Maryland, which has had a good Family Life and Human Development curriculum for many years—are fully supported by students and parents. Parents have an option not to permit their children to take these sex education courses. Over the years thousands of students have been sex-educated, with less than *2 percent* of the parents opting to remove their children from these classes. Where is all this massive opposition to our type of sex-education that groups including the John Birch Society, Moral Majority, Concerned Women for America, Citizens for Excellence in Education, Family Research Council, Focus on the Family, Traditional Values Coalition, and the Christian Coalition are trying to persuade the American public exists?

The antis are not above outrageous lies. For a while they circulated the spurious story that a female teacher undressed in front of her sex education class in order to make the course relevant. A "book burning" team in West Virginia stated that our book *Facts About Sex for Today's Youth* had explicit drawings of sexual positions. We looked again and couldn't find any. Another critic described our work as the "glorification of immodesty, impurity and sexual permissiveness" and went on to say that our views can be expressed as follows: "Any form of sexual expression is 'healthy' and 'moral' if pleasurable, hygienic and voluntary."

Of course, this critic left out words that we *do* use, such as "adult," "mature," "nonexploitive," "guilt-free," "enhancing of the person," "consenting." The most frequent accusation leveled at sex educators is that they preach to teenagers, "If it feels good, do it." This is an absurd fabrication, and we know of no sex educator who endorses that position for young people—or adults, for that matter.

Another leading opponent of sex education described our publications in the following manner:

> I believe they're right. It's educational. But what are they educating them for? If gals want to grow up to run a house of prostitution, they know exactly what supplies are needed. I think it's a demoralizing promotion by Communism. If they get the young people interested in sex, they can demoralize the country and just walk in and take it over. That's the Communist procedure.

If you are not convinced that the anti–sex educators are well organized and serious, read this quote from a strategy pamphlet that has been widely circulated among them:

> [Go] to school board meetings in your town and other towns—applaud and groan at the right times and, if necessary, stomp your feet and scream. The more brazen you are, the more attention you'll get. Don't refer to school programs as family life and sex education but simply call them sex pro-

grams. It'll upset them and, when they're upset, they don't think as well.

Parents and society in general would be wise to keep in mind the admonition of the eighteenth-century Jewish sage Baal Shem-Tov, who said, "The world is full of people who in the guise of piety are ready to harass others."

More sober opponents like to cite statistics that "prove" that sex education programs in the United States and elsewhere have failed to discourage irresponsible sexual behavior among the young. Generally they make the mistake of lumping together both optimal and inadequate programs and then drawing sweeping conclusions based on the faulty evidence. Nevertheless, a good general principle is: *Don't overstate the value of sex education in the schools.* It can transmit information, reduce sex-related guilt, foster a sense of responsibility, and even reduce rates of unintended pregnancies and STDs by 10 to 20 percent over a five- to ten-year period. But, without reducing the most compelling reasons for teen pregnancy, namely, poor school performance, racism, sexism, poverty, and individual vulnerability, officials should not hope for overwhelming success.

In addition, programs conducted in schools where there are big discipline problems and low morale certainly can't be expected to have good results. Such courses would simply have no credibility in the eyes of the students.

What a pity that we still must share the view of the author of a book about sex education in Britain (*My Mother Said...The Way Young People Learned About Sex and Birth Control,* by Christine Farrell): that neither males nor females are "currently given as much information as they would wish for, at an age they think appropriate, or from a source which they regard as authoritative." The biggest source of information is 6 to 8 hours per day of TV and rock music.

There is concern among some parents that sex educators are attempting to replace parents as the primary sex educators of children. There is simply no basis for this fear. Even the best, most comprehensive sex education program seeks only to supplement the primary responsibilities of parents. The schools, religions, and governmental agencies all have a secondary role in providing information and services for young people; the *primary* responsibility for sex-educating children from birth to adulthood always has been and must remain in the home. Parents provide the love, warmth, and caring that are the foundations of many future values and attitudes concerning sexuality, and family life can only be strengthened by parents who take an active role in communicating with their own children.

The Case for a Moral Sex Education

F *irst we must make the case* for a moral education in the public schools. "Our liberal democratic heritage expressed in the American constitutional framework of secular limited government is our strongest bulwark for personal liberty and human rights," says Edward L. Ericson, in *American Freedom and the Radical Right.* "True moral democracy...is always a morality of diversity, liberty and civil tolerance."

As Aristotle suggested, people do not naturally grow up to be morally excellent. They become so only as a result of a lifelong personal and community effort.

Human beings are not necessarily born with a capacity for behaving democratically or altruistically. Moral development takes place within a community of persons; any individual's sense of right and wrong develops in interaction with others. For one individual to impose dogmatically his or her point of view on another would interfere with moral development and individual liberty.

There is a vast difference between being moral and being moralistic. Moralistic stances leave little room for dissent and dialogue.

For example, a teacher could state that it is a health hazard for young people to smoke. This is a statement of fact as well as a moral position. It would be moralistic for the teacher to declare, "It is a sin to smoke." Moralistic statements clearly are inappropriate for public schools.[1]

The tension between one person's liberty and another's is a moral issue. Put another way, a central moral dilemma is, how can I exercise my individual liberty without harming another person or myself? Or, how can I exercise my individual liberty and enhance the growth of another?

Young people need to understand these complex issues. They need to learn how to apply moral principles to situations in their own lives. The community—that is, parents, teachers, and clergy—has the responsibility to help young people. If principles are imposed with no room for discussion and working through, then the possibility of developing into a morally excellent person is prematurely foreclosed.

If, at its heart, education is moral education, then we have to face the fact that values will be part of the process. Education cannot be conducted in a value-free context.

In social studies, for example, the teacher doesn't say, "All forms of government are equally good. Choose one." The teacher explains that democracy is what the founding American fathers thought was best. Democracy, in their understanding, offers the maximum benefits to the most people and protects them from exploitation. The notion of democracy, then, is value-laden. The Constitution guarantees the right to life, liberty, and the pursuit of happiness. Laws protect us from persons who interfere with these rights.

Moral education would foster the basic values embodied in the Bill of Rights. Since America is a democratic society, and public

---

1. Cf. article in the *New York Times*—"High Schools Tackle Marital Skills, Igniting Debate," Oct. 14, 1998, p. B9.

schools are committed to these values, moral education is logical and appropriate for American society. The basic principle of a moral education is the democratic principle of human equality. In practice, it is difficult to apply, but it provides a goal toward which educators can help students strive.

The values to be taught, then, are the values of democratic society. They are not static in some of their applications: the Constitution is amended from time to time. The essence of these values, however, is considered universal and unchanging over time. The concept of community standards, so often applied to controversies at the local level in regard to racial or sexual matters, needs to be examined carefully when designing a moral education. Racist attitudes did, and in some ways still do, reflect community standards in sections of our country. It is wrong to preach or practice racism in the schools, though useful to teach about its history.

In moral education, however, we teach the highest aspirations of our society, no matter what is manifested in isolated locales or in the pronouncements of extremist groups. Equality of the sexes, dignity, and respect for all human beings, regardless of their race, religion, sexual orientation, or country of origin, all stem from the fundamental democratic premise of equality.

In this context, all controversial issues can be discussed, even such volatile issues as abortion and masturbation. To teach a controversial issue, one must, fairly and rationally, present a range of points of view without exaggeration and in keeping with a scientific perspective.

Proselytizing in the public schools violates our constitutional rights and liberties. In this country we are firmly committed to separation of church and state. Of course we endorse a value-laden, moral education, but whose values? Ours. The moral aspirations of the democratic society in which we live. We are opposed to racism, sexism, and the double standard. We favor equal opportunities for men and women. We're opposed to rape and sexual exploitation of children.

It's not difficult to make a distinction between using good judgment and being judgmental. We are, after all, a democratic society, dedicated to diversity of opinion and religious beliefs. We're clear that the ideal is to have justice that is not influenced by race, religion, and gender. We are not naive; though life is not fair, we aim to create fairness through the justice system.

Although American society subscribes to the principle of equality, in practice the poor, blacks, the disabled, women, and children are often exceptions. There are many other ways to damage the dignity of others, e.g., coercion. Intimidation can involve physical aggression or threats, or it can play upon another person's sense of self. The classic words of coercion in male–female relationships are, "You would if you loved me." Exposure to moral education mitigates against exploitation in the guise of seduction and demonstrates how moral development would be enhanced by teaching a full range of these ideas.

Some school systems are now teaching moral values. The Salt Lake City School district, for example, has introduced moral education into its curriculum. Some of their basic principles illustrate how democratic values can be an explicit part of the curriculum with time set aside for student discussion. Here are some of the principles:

1. Each individual has dignity and worth.
2. A free society requires respect for all persons, property, and principles.
3. Each person is responsible for his or her own actions.
4. Each individual has a responsibility to the group as well as to the total society.

Mary S. Calderone and Eric Johnson (*The Family Book About Sexuality*), both preoccupied with the moral dimensions of sexuality, developed a perspective that is useful for our purpose. They suggest that the following six values should be acceptable in our American democracy:

The Case for a Moral Sex Education

1. The value of information
2. The value of responsibility
3. The value of control
4. The value of consideration
5. The value of each individual person
6. The value of communication

We firmly endorse the position approved by the Values Education Commission of the Maryland State Department of Education, July 30, 1979:

> ...the Commission takes the view that the public schools are appropriate, indeed necessary, institutions in a democratic society for defining and encouraging character and citizenship values. The schools cannot supplant the role played by the family and religion in values education, but they can reinforce positive attitudes and behavior and counteract negative influences on the students.

The Commission recognizes that responsible personal and citizenship behavior can be encouraged by the entire public school experience as well as by special efforts within the curriculum to deal with the rights and duties of citizens in a democracy.

CHARACTER OBJECTIVES

1. Personal integrity and honesty rooted in respect for the truth, intellectual curiosity, and love of learning.
2. A sense of duty to self, family, school, and community.
3. Self-esteem rooted in the recognition of one's potential.
4. Respect for the rights of all persons regardless of their race, religion, sex, age, physical condition, or mental state. (We would add "sexual orientation" here.)

5. A recognition of the right of others to hold and express differing views, combined with the capacity to make discriminating judgments among competing opinions.
6. A sense of justice, rectitude, fair play, and a commitment to them.
7. A disposition of understanding, sympathy, concern, and compassion for others.
8. A sense of discipline and pride in one's work; respect for the achievements of others.
9. Respect for one's property and the property of others, including public property.
10. Courage to express one's convictions.

CITIZENSHIP OBJECTIVES

1. Patriotism: love, respect, and loyalty to the United States of America and the willingness to correct its imperfections by legal means.
2. An understanding of the rights and obligations of a citizen in a democratic society
3. An understanding of other societies in the world which do not enjoy the rights and privileges of a democratic government. (We are not sure about this one. In our judgment, we should not support cruel dictatorships.)
4. Respect for the U.S. Constitution, the rule of law, and the right of every citizen to enjoy equality under the law. An understanding of the Bill of Rights and a recognition that all rights are limited by other rights and by obligations. Respect for legitimate authority at the local, state, and federal levels.
5. Allegiance to the concept of democratic government as opposed to totalitarian rule. A recognition that government is limited by the separation of powers and by the countervailing role of other institutions in a pluralistic society—principally the family, religion, the school, and the private sector of the economy.

6. Recognition of the need for an independent court system to protect the rights of all citizens.
7. An acceptance of all citizenship responsibilities at the local, state, and national levels and a commitment to preserve and defend the United States and its democratic institutions.

John Dewey suggested in the late 1800s that schools should focus less on what to do and more on "how to decide what to do."

Dewey opposed moral instructions that relied heavily on oaths, creeds, codes, prayers, and extrinsic rewards. In order to facilitate moral development, Dewey suggested, schools should provide opportunities in cooperation, self-direction, and leadership, rather than conformity, passivity, and blind submission to authority.

The majority of Americans favor sex education in the schools, according to all polls. Yet less than 10 percent of American school-children are exposed to anything approaching a good sex education. All you need is three or four opponents in almost any community and the sex education program is finished, because school boards are overly responsive to these extremists. Fortunately, after a long, hard struggle this did not turn out to be the case in New Jersey, where sex education is now mandated. As of 1998, only about twenty states have a statewide mandate to teach reasonably good sexuality education. There continue to be attacks on these mandates both federally and at the state level.

Opponents of sex education want you to believe that if you tell kids about sex, they'll do it. All our research reveals that young people who are knowledgeable about their sexuality are more likely to delay their first sexual experience. **KNOWLEDGE IS NOT HARMFUL.** Virtually all opposition in this country to sex education is based on the supposition that knowledge is harmful.

Let me conclude by telling you a true story that represents the value of values. A young college student came to me absolutely in despair and said, "Listen, my boyfriend and I took your course and we plan to get married, but our marriage is threatened because he wants to have sex before marriage and I don't. I don't care if I'm the last virgin. I want to be a virgin on my wedding night. We had such a fight that we decided to compromise. We will leave it up to Dr. Gordon to decide."

Now, if I were a modern psychologist I would say, "Listen, I can't tell you what to do, you need therapy. At the end I still won't be able to tell you what to do, because I can't impose my values on you. You'll develop a little insight and you'll figure out what to do." I didn't say that. I said, "Listen, if you have sex with him under those circumstances, you're stupid." She was thrilled, but wanted to know what she should tell him. I said to tell him that if he really loved her he wouldn't put this kind of pressure on her. She said, "Oh my God, that never occurred to me." (A college senior, yet.) She went home to talk to her boyfriend. A half-hour later she called and said, "I told him." What did he say? "He said you have a point."

CHAPTER SEVEN

What Children Need to Know: The Preschool and Preteen Years

I*n a questionnaire given* to 450 Syracuse University undergraduates, more than 50 percent thought that their parents were comfortable with their own sexuality. But, when asked "As you were growing up, what would you wish your parents had told you about sex?", about 90 percent of these same students indicated that sex was not honestly discussed in their homes.

- "I wish my parents had canned the stork story and fairy tale explanations—and told me the truth."
- "I wish my parents sat me down and told me about sex instead of just saying, 'don't let no one in your pants.'"
- "I wish that my parents had talked to me about sex—going beyond menstruation, pubic hair, etc."
- "I wish my parents had been more open about sex and not treated it as a big dark secret to be discovered and experienced after marriage."
- "I wish they had told me not to feel so inhibited about my body. I wish they told me that there was nothing wrong with making love with someone if it is right and special."

- "I wish my parents spoke to me more about birth control and let me know that in trouble I could turn to them."
- "I wish Mom had told me that first sexual encounters—meaning intercourse, per se—would probably be fairly disappointing in most ways."

Only about 10 percent of the students seemed to be satisfied with their parents' efforts or nonefforts at sex education.

The clearest message to emerge from our work in sexuality education is that children appreciate openness and candor at an early age. Parents who rarely communicate with their children when young have the most difficulty talking with teenagers, whom they finally perceive as being old enough to understand. Often the credibility of parents is diminished when they give the impression that any area *except* human sexuality is open for discussion.

It might be instructive to know a little about how one of us—Sol Gordon—got into this field. I was working in a child-guidance clinic at a time when sexuality was not much discussed. This was no accident, because virtually no medical school or professional school of psychology, social work, or nursing included courses in sexuality at that time. Thus, doctors and other professionals who were supposed to know the most often didn't know any more than the people who were asking the questions. This amounted to a conspiracy of silence, even in the heyday of psychoanalysis when sex was assumed to be the root of all neurosis.

Under the circumstances, any discussion was so abstract that it didn't help average people understand their own sexuality, their children's sexuality, or some of the conflicts between the two. Practical questions regarding such topics as penis or vagina size, the clitoris, the role of communication in sexual functioning, and a host of others went unanswered.

Once, as part of a study, we asked one hundred teenagers (fifty boys and fifty girls) if their parents had talked to them about sex. Each one said no. Then we asked the parents if they had spoken to their children about this subject. All said that they had in fact done so. These contradictory results were fascinating because one seldom gets such widely divergent findings. We pursued the matter eagerly, asking the teenagers if they really couldn't remember or perhaps weren't telling the truth. When we pushed the teenagers harder still, virtually all of the girls remembered that their mothers had talked to them about menstruation. The rest of the communication could be summed up in one word: **Don't.** The boys were less impressed by our efforts to jog their memories. However, once we spoke of the ritual of "going out for a walk," about half of the boys remembered it taking place when they were about eleven years old. We decided they remembered an awkward discussion about the birds and the bees, both father and son so embarrassed that very little real communication took place. Some did recall the father ending the conversation with the remark that if worse came to worse, the son could always find some condoms in the father's drawer.

This research is forty years old now, but it still seems to contain elements of truth. Whenever large mixed adult audiences are told about it, there is nervous laughter suggesting that perhaps it had been part of their own experience. Their reaction reinforces our strong belief that sex should more than a single or occasional talk, connected only to significant physical developments in a child's life. Sexuality education should be an **ongoing process.** Becoming an askable parent starts *long* before the child goes to school. The parent who has discussed sexuality openly with the young child can expect the teenager to share confidences later.

Parents need to understand what experiences affect children in their early years, especially if they are to help them develop positive attitudes toward themselves and others. In this light, we'd like to share with readers a letter we received from a mother who feared that she and her husband were not very successful in their efforts to help and guide their children. The letter highlights a dilemma that is faced by all parents, and that demands that we be realistic in our appraisal of parent–child relationships.

It may sound strange to other people when we say this, but my husband and I know that we have been good parents. We've raised our children firmly but lovingly, have made sure they know what our values are, and have given them a good sex education. Thus, it disturbs me tremendously when our children behave in ways that contradict so strongly what we've taught them. For instance, our 10-year-old son insists on calling some of his friends "faggot," even though we've told him many times that this is offensive. My husband and I wind up looking at each other and saying, "He didn't get it from us,"—but where do these things come from?

Our answer:

Your question illustrates so well how outside influences sometimes overwhelm even our best intentions. We can guide our children, but we can't exercise full control over them. A good approach is to make sure that children know the meaning of the derogatory words they're using. Then focus on your own attitude rather than criticizing them. For example, get across the message that you would appreciate it if they wouldn't use such terms, and you would feel much better if they were a bit more sensitive on this subject. Ask the children to think through how they would feel if their friend or sibling really were a homosexual.

Such incidents should not be the occasion for parental self-doubt or feelings of failure. The effects of talking openly about sexuality and other important topics may not be immediately apparent, but these things have a way of taking hold, provided that we're not too impatient. As Lisa Strick said in an article in *Woman's Day*: "Talking about sex at home—openly and truthfully—won't guarantee that your children will be virgins when they marry. But it might prevent them from becoming parents before they've had a chance to find out what it is to be grown up."

WHAT YOU NEED TO KNOW
ABOUT INFANTILE SEXUALITY

Sexual pleasure is not confined to stimulation of the genitals, nor is all pleasant physical contact related to sex. This is true even of the youngest of babies, who learn about the pleasures of physical contact through loving fondling. Parents stroke, kiss, and cuddle their babies, and the babies respond with affection. They find great satisfaction in using their mouths when eating and when sucking on the toes or other objects.

An infant is learning even though he or she does not yet talk. The infant will use this early learning later in life. What infants learn about love, affection, and physical contact will affect their sexual attitudes and behaviors when they become biologically ready to have children, in the period called puberty. Many of a person's sexual feelings and attitudes are determined before the age of five.

For instance, toilet-training before children are ready can create feelings of self-doubt, guilt, and shame. These feelings may trouble the youngsters for the rest of their lives, though they probably won't even be aware of them. Suppose that a child has an "accident" and is punished, or simply is told that he or she is "bad" or "dirty." If the child is not capable or old enough to control elimination, he or she may become (honestly) confused and develop serious feelings of anxiety, guilt, and inferiority.

Children need to be handled with patience and understanding. This means that parents must stop and think. Can you imagine what the child is feeling and help him see it? Can you treat her firmly and kindly at the same time? Explore alternatives to punishing. Share with others.

This applies as well to infants beginning to discover and explore their bodies. If parents slap a child's fingers or pull the hand away for playing with the genitals even though they coo and smile and comment on how cute the child looks when playing with his or her toes, the child will be confused and may associate the genitals with feelings of guilt and shame.

No one expects babies who are barely old enough to walk, talk, or know where the bathroom is to be anything but innocent and carefree. Only when children are old enough to go to the bathroom on their own can parents teach them the difference between public and private behavior.

We have already discussed such issues as masturbation, nudity in the home, and obscenities (see Chapter 4, "Becoming an Askable Parent"). Treating the child's developing growth and awareness in these areas with respect and acceptance is perhaps more important in the early years of life than at any other time.

Sometimes we forget the fact that sexuality is something we *are* rather than something we *do*. When a baby is born, we often ask, "What is it? Is it a boy or a girl?" We then program children according to sex as they get older. It may be less popular these days for children to be identified in terms of dress—blue for boys and pink for girls—but stereotyping remains a fact of life for many youngsters. Remarks like "That's not for a boy," "Act like a man!" and "That's not ladylike!" are still common in some families. Boys and girls get the impression that nothing is more terrible than "acting" like a member of the opposite sex.

The following letter from a mother demonstrates how volatile an issue this can become in some homes.

My husband and I have strong differences of opinion about our four-year-old son who occasionally likes to play house with his girlfriends. He seems to be a big disappointment to my husband because of his apparent lack of interest in so-called "male" activities such as playing with trucks and guns. I'm sure that in the back of my husband's mind is the idea that if we don't discourage our son's "effeminate" activities now, he'll become a homosexual later on.

Our answer:

It is always difficult when parents disagree. You might want to tell your husband that the more he criticizes your son's behavior, the more unhappy your son will become, not the more masculine. The very best approach would be for him to make it a point to spend time with the child alone, slowly and gradually involving him in activities that your husband finds more appropriate. There is no real substitute for working on an improved relationship between father and son first, before focusing on the specific "problems" of your son.

Parents do worry about sexual confusion and sexual identity. Even "liberal" parents can become concerned when their little boys appear to enjoy dressing up in women's clothing. There is somewhat less concern for girls who take on "tomboyish" traits. Most often, but not necessarily, such behavior is a transitional stage and nothing more. Our advice is to test it out and see if not "fussing" makes other interests become predominant. Should these cross-sexual traits maintain themselves over a long period of time, they may indicate gender confusion. Yet one should be concerned only if they seem to reflect a basic neurotic trend in the development of the child, a trend symptomatic of other areas of maladjustment. A child who makes friends, enjoys life, and, at the same time, takes on the so-called sensitivity of the opposite sex (even in terms of the popular stereotypes) may be evidencing a background for creativity and good emotional development. Our advice is to be concerned only if other behaviors such as bedwetting, not eating or sleeping, extreme introversion, and a general disorganization of the personality persist. Things have changed since we were kids, making it easier for us as parents. Some girls love athletic games, while some boys concentrate on music and theater.

Why do parents need to think about these questions before they arise? For one thing, they're in the media every day and references are heard at school often. Such thought is an investment in prevention! Even the most sophisticated and alert parents can get confused when confronted by their children at unexpected moments with such questions as "Where did I come from?" and "How did I get into you?" Parents can prepare their responses beforehand. Farther on in this chapter we list a number of questions typical of preschool children along with our suggested responses.

You may feel that a child's question is inappropriate at that moment, but the very fact that the child asked it indicates its appropriateness from his or her perspective. A child should never be given the impression that he or she has asked the wrong question, that the timing is wrong, or that there is something wrong with the child for asking the question in the first place. Parents may prefer that everything be done according to their expectations, in line with certain developmental stages or at points when they personally feel ready, but children are full of surprises. That's part of the excitement of raising children.

SOME PARENTAL CONCERNS

There are some specific sexually related questions or situations about which parents may be concerned. For example, how should you react to a child who wants to climb into bed with you? We feel that this is okay. Many adults recall that some of their most pleasant experiences took place early in childhood when they could have a lot of fun with their parents in bed. Some parents worry about sexual stimulation, but most are quite comfortable with the idea. Even if they find themselves becoming stimulated by this contact, they are able to acknowledge the sensual delight of loving their children so closely. The natural warmth between parents and children provides children with a sound basis for their later capacity to love and be loving parents themselves. It is usually playful rather than erotic.

On the other hand, we don't think it is good policy to allow children to sleep with parents. If your child has traumatic dreams or nightmares and wants the comfort of sleeping with you, it might be a good idea to say, "I'll stay with you for a while until you fall asleep." Or to invite the child to come to your bed for a while until comforted, then carry the youngster back to bed.

It is quite common for children to have upsetting nightmares, and one shouldn't dismiss the experience by simply telling them not to worry about it. Parents can tell children that they know nightmares are frightening and that everyone has them at one time or another. The important thing is to reassure them that all they have to do is open their eyes and the nightmare will disappear.

We share parental concerns about television, not because of the exposure to sexual information (as opposed to pornography, sarcasm, and cynicism) but because of the violence, including abusive and exploitive relationships and teasing. It is wise for parents to set television watching limits and make sure that it is not used as a substitute for activity, learning, and achieving.

The elementary school age is the time for developing basic academic skills and establishing good study habits. The old notion that this constitutes a "latency" period when children are not particularly interested in anything sexual is a myth perpetuated by Freudian diehards. We've rarely met children of school age who were not aware and excited, interested in, and affected by the sexual aspects of their lives. They'll ask questions and be curious. They'll certainly observe what's happening on television. They'll notice pregnancies and they'll wonder where the puppies next door came from. This is a good age to respond candidly and freely to all pertinent sexually oriented questions. (It is not appropriate to answer questions about your own private sexual life.)

SEXUAL ABUSE OF CHILDREN

This is a painful and difficult issue: sexual molestation of children. Sexual abuse may occur to children of any age, from infants through the teenage years. (The most common age is from eleven to fourteen years old.) A realistic understanding of molestation is essential for parents, particularly since this area has been clouded by misinformation and taboos.

The National Center on Child Abuse and Neglect has estimated that of the one million child-abuse cases reported each year, 12 percent were victims of sexual molestation. Most were girls abused by fathers, stepfathers, and close relatives.

Child molestation crosses all social, economic, and racial boundaries and affects a wide range of family situations. Stereotypes that portray the offenders as obviously neurotic, lecherous, "dirty old men," even psychotic, are inaccurate. The phenomenon does usually seem to be accompanied by manifestations of low self-esteem and of self-destructive behavior. Incest can continue only in secret, and the families involved are typically isolated from friends and the mainstream of life.

We strongly recommend that parents of young children read to them our book entitled *A Better Safe Than Sorry Book: A Family Guide for Sexual Assault Prevention.* (See Recommended Books.)

The Federal Child Abuse Prevention and Treatment Act defines child abuse, including sexual abuse or exploitation, as injury or maltreatment of a child "by a person who is responsible for the child's welfare." The National Center of Child Abuse and Neglect has adopted a broader definition:

...contacts or interactions between a child and an adult when the child is being used for the sexual stimulation of the perpetrator or another person. Sexual abuse may also be committed by a person under the age of 18 when that person is either significantly older than the victim or when the perpetrator is in a position of power or control over another child.

The very nature of the power relationship between parents or other adults and children often inhibits the youngsters from revealing the sexual advances made against them. Subtle or overt threats are often made to discourage exposing the situation.

Sometimes the child is sufficiently sophisticated to perceive some of the possible consequences: loss of family income, police or social-service intervention and subsequent court trials, psychiatric treatment or incarceration, the breakup of the family, and public shame. Once in the open, the situation must be handled sensitively for the child's sake; interviews, medical examinations, and court procedures must be conducted with an awareness of the child's acute fears and anxieties.

Not long ago a close friend of ours from the Midwest called one evening in a near-hysterical state; her twelve-year-old daughter had been approached sexually by her grandfather, the woman's father. The grandfather, as is often the case, was a responsible member of the community, a proverbial "pillar" of family rectitude. The child's experience had triggered a memory the mother had long repressed: when she was the same age as her daughter, her father had sexually molested her. As a young teenager, she had dealt with it fairly well, told no one, and repressed the incident altogether. Though she had managed reasonably well to overcome her feelings of fear and guilt, in retrospect she realized that it had inhibited her sexual responsiveness and healthy adjustment to adulthood. When she confronted her father with the truth, he denied it absolutely and acted as if she had imagined the whole thing. Her own mother accused her of hating her father and plotting to destroy the family.

These reactions are not atypical; only a fraction of child-molestation incidents are brought to the attention of authorities, and even fewer are successfully prosecuted. In truth, no absolute guidelines can be set for the disposition of such cases. Not all should be dealt with outside the context of the family or come under legal jurisdiction. We are, however, convinced that being molested is most often a traumatizing experience for the child involved, even though most recover with strong support.

Once upon a time, a parent's precaution was simply to tell a child never to accept candy or rides from a stranger. But strangers, as modern statistics point out, represent only about 25 percent of the offenders (to be sure, when it does involve a stranger, enticements are usually involved). Parents as well as caretakers need to convey a somewhat different message to children. They should tell them that no one—stranger, neighbor, relative, or family member—has the right to touch or fondle their genitals. The child should understand that even if it is someone he or she knows and loves, it is still not right.

Generally speaking, the message to the child might be: "If someone ever touches you there or asks or forces you to touch them, please tell us right away. Say no and get away if you can. Even if the person makes you promise not to tell anyone, that is a promise you should not keep. If you are threatened or forced to do things, you may have to go along with them, but even if you 'swear to God' not to tell your mother, God doesn't expect you to keep promises that hurt you. Whenever someone says, 'Don't tell your mother,' that's a good way of knowing that whatever they are asking you to do is wrong." Children can be told these things without being caused excessive alarm or scared unduly.

Relatives as well as the victims themselves often develop a keen desire for revenge and punishment for the molester. But jail and retribution are rarely as rehabilitative as counseling and therapy can be. Child-abuse hotlines and special counseling centers now exist in every state. They offer support, counseling, referrals, and legal assistance to victims as well as victimizers. With more than eight hundred chapters nationwide, Parents Anonymous (PA) is a major resource: (909) 621-6184.

Recently, some researchers have suggested that the pain and trauma associated with incidents of child molestation have been exaggerated. Yet few, if any, victims have come forward to declare that they benefited from the experiences. The absence of trauma is hardly evidence of a positive effect; many victims survive the experience without suffering terribly, but others later have enormous feelings of guilt, anger, and outrage.

If a child informs a parent that he or she has been sexually molested, there are things the parent can do to help alleviate the child's suffering. First (and this will be difficult), try to control your own anxiety level. If the child senses that you are devastated by the situation, it could magnify the child's own misery. Parents should never say things like "Why did you let him do it?" or "Why didn't you run away?" Such questions imply that the incident was somehow the child's fault. We want to state unequivocally that it is *always* the responsibility of the molester. No matter how "seductive" or "flirtatious" a little girl might seem, she is not to be blamed for an adult male's inability to control his impulses.

Perhaps most importantly, comfort the child. Let her know that you still love and value her. The child may appear fearful for a time afterward and may need immense reassurance of her continuing worth, safety, and acceptance in the family. How the child reacts largely depends on how the family responds to the situation. (Our *A Better Safe Than Sorry Book* is designed for children aged three to nine.)

PRETEENS

There are two areas where parents must accept responsibility: preparing girls for the onset of menstruation and preparing boys for nocturnal emissions. These talks should occur well in advance so the events are not traumatic surprises. Girls should also know about nocturnal emissions, just as boys should be told about menstruation.

When a girl is nine or ten, her mother or female relative can demonstrate the proper method of using sanitary napkins or tampons. This is the time to give a positive explanation of menstruation as a normal and healthy bodily process experienced by all females, starting around eleven to fifteen years old. It is a positive step in her physical development, the beginning of maturity.

At the same age, boys can be told by either parent or a relative about wet dreams, which happen to most boys and are a normal stage of male development, starting somewhere between eleven and fifteen years of age. Let him know that his linens may get wet and that he can put them in the hamper if this happens. Wet dreams are related to sexual impulses and thoughts and will occur less frequently as he gets older. By the time there are opportunities for regular sexual outlets, they are likely to cease.

IN THEIR OWN WORDS

Children under six often ask very good questions. Here are some, along with suggested responses.

• *Where did I come from?*
You began in a special place inside Mommy called the uterus. When you were ready to be born, you came out through Mommy's vagina. Both Mommy and Daddy were needed to get you started.

• *How did I get inside you?*
When Daddy and I felt very cuddly in bed, Daddy put his penis into my vagina. A tiny seed called a sperm from Daddy met a tiny egg called an ovum inside me. That's how you got started. You were so small that I wasn't sure at first if a baby was beginning to grow inside me. You grew and grew in my uterus for a long time. Then you were born.

• *Where was I before I got inside you?*
You weren't anywhere. Daddy and I got you started. When I felt you growing inside, we were very happy.

• *How long did I have to grow until you saw me?*
It took nine months for you to grow in my uterus before you were born. But I knew that you were there. You began kicking when you had been in my uterus only around five months. You didn't kick hard, just enough to let me know that you were there and to say, "Hi." I also grew very big in front.

• *Why does Jim have a penis and I don't?*
That's one of the differences between boys and girls. Girls have a vagina and boys don't. Only girls have a vulva. Do you know what part of you is called the vulva? Do you know where your vagina is?

• *A three-year-old boy taking a shower with his dad wants to know, "Why is your penis bigger than mine?"*
As you get older, your penis will become larger and be like mine.

• *A four-year-old girl taking a shower with her mother points to the mother's breasts and asks, "How come you have two and I don't have any?"*
As you grow older, you will develop breasts, too.

• *How do babies get food before they are born?*
Every time the mother eats something, the baby gets a little of that food. Also, every time the mother breathes, the baby receives a little oxygen.

• *Did you know that I would be a girl before I was born?*
No, mothers and fathers do not usually know that. They know that they are going to have a baby. When the baby is born, if it has a vagina, it's a girl. If it has a penis, it's a boy. There are special ways of finding out the baby's sex before birth, but most parents prefer the surprise.

• *Five-year-old Eddie is having a bath with his four-year-old sister, Suzy. She notices that Eddie's penis is hard and sticking straight out. She asks her mother why.*
Eddie has what is called an erection. This happens to all boys occasionally. It's a nice feeling when it happens.

• *Does it hurt to have a baby?*
Yes, having a baby does hurt. Do you remember when you fell and bumped your head? It hurt for just a little while and then

you forgot about it. It's the same thing when you have a baby. It usually hurts only a little while.

• *Why can't I sleep with you?*
Because Daddy and I sleep in the same bed. We like privacy at night. (Single parents can just say they prefer sleeping by themselves.)

• *What's privacy?*
Privacy means that you want to be alone sometimes. Occasionally, two people like Mommy and Daddy enjoy being together without anyone else there. You, too, want to be by yourself at times. Then you can sing and play and no one will disturb you.

• *Aunt Jackie doesn't feed Baby Alice from her breast. How come?*
Because Aunt Jackie decided that she would rather feed Baby Alice from a bottle. Every mother makes her own decision about that.

• *Mom, will you tell Emily where babies come from? Her mom won't tell her. Her mom said those things were dirty and she shouldn't ask questions.*
That's too bad. You and I know that isn't so. I don't think that there are any dirty questions. I want you to ask me anything you want to know. I'll try to answer. I hope that Emily's mom in time will talk to her in the same way you and I are talking now.

• *Whom do you love most, Daddy or me?*
I love each of you differently. I love Grandma and Grandpa differently also. There are many kinds of love.

• *Can I love myself?*
When you look into the mirror and smile at yourself, or when you feel good about you, then you love yourself. It's very important that you love yourself, because then it will be easier for you to love others and for others to love you.

IN THEIR OWN WORDS

Children who are six, seven, eight, or almost nine might have questions like these:

• *Does every woman have a baby?*
No, not every woman has a baby. Women who have sexual intercourse with men can have babies. When a seed called a sperm from a man comes together with an egg called an ovum from a woman, a baby gets started.

Not every woman wants to have a baby. Most who do want children are having smaller families these days. We can use special things called contraceptives if we want to have intercourse without making a baby.

• *What are contraceptives?*
Mommy and Daddy have sex because we enjoy it. It's one of the nice things grown-ups do. When we are not trying to have a baby, we use a special method that keeps Mommy from getting pregnant. Pregnant means that a woman is going to have a baby.

• *How old is grown up?*
A lot of people think that grown up is when you are over eighteen years old or when you get married.

• *Can I have a baby now and can Jimmy be its daddy?*
You can start having babies only after you start to menstruate. But you should not have a baby until you can take care of it. Jimmy is also not ready. It's better to wait until you are grown up and married.

• *What's a tampon for?*
Girls and women use a tampon when they are menstruating in order to protect their clothing.

Raising a Child Responsibly in a Sexually Permissive World

• *Do I have to be married to have children?*
It would be better for the baby if you and the baby's father were married. It's very hard to bring up children by yourself. It can be done—some people do it. When you are older, you'll want to decide many things about your future. One of these things will be which job you want. Another will be where you want to live, and still another will be if you want to get married and have children. You will have lots of time to think about those things.

• *How does a baby get out of a mommy's tummy?*
First of all, the baby is not in Mommy's tummy. I know it looks that way to you. A baby rests in a special place called the uterus. When it is ready to be born, it comes out through the vagina. The vagina doesn't seem big enough, but it stretches so the baby can come out.

Most babies are born this way, but not all. When a mother is having trouble giving birth to a baby, doctors sometimes perform an operation called a Caesarean section. This is a simple surgical technique. Doctors make an incision—a cut—in the mother's lower abdomen. Then they remove the baby from the uterus. It doesn't take long, and the baby isn't hurt by it. The mother heals quickly and is back on her feet within a few days. Many mothers have this operation, and children born this way are just like any others.

• *How does a baby get started?*
Before a man and a woman have sexual intercourse, they lie together making love. During that time the man's penis hardens and the woman's vagina lubricates. The man puts his penis into the woman's vagina when she feels ready. After a little while sperm comes out of the man's penis. If sperm unite with an ovum in the woman's uterus, a baby gets started.

• *What is a prostitute?*
A prostitute is a person who is willing to have sexual relations for money. It is not legal in our country, but it happens.

• *What are the main differences between men and women?*
The main differences show up in most girls after they are twelve and boys after they are thirteen. Women can have babies. Women's breasts develop and they can breast-feed their babies. Women menstruate. Men can father children with the sperm made in their testicles.

As we think about it, men and women are more alike than different. Most men and women want to have a good education, find a job they like, have time for fun, make friends, fall in love with someone they would like to marry, have a nice family, and be good citizens of the country in which they live.

• *How can a woman know if she's pregnant?*
In order for a conception to occur, sexual intercourse has to have taken place. (Exceptions are pregnancies produced by artificial insemination, in vitro fertilization, and accidental entry of sperm ejaculated near the vagina.) A girl can get pregnant from having had intercourse only once. She will not have her menstrual period, although there can be some spotting. Usually, her breasts become tender and slightly enlarged. Often she will feel nauseated and may vomit, especially in the morning. She will gain a little weight at the beginning. Some women have all of these signs right away, some have only one or two of them, some none. Any of these symptoms must be considered significant, and, if they occur, a pregnancy test should be done, preferably in a doctor's office.

• *What is incest?*
Incest occurs when two people who are closely related have sexual relations. It could be a father and daughter, a mother and son, or a brother and sister. Incest is illegal; both government and religion have forbidden incestuous relationships.

Children cannot marry parents, brothers and sisters cannot marry each other, and in many states cousins are also not allowed to marry. When they get older, most people meet and fall in love with someone they are not related to.

• *What is oral sex?*
When the mouth is placed on the genitals for sexual pleasure. Some people like it. Some people don't.

• *What is anal sex?*
When the penis enters the anus for sexual pleasure. Some people like it. Some people don't. Because of the danger of STD—especially AIDS—it should never be tried without using a condom.

IN OUR WORDS

Here are some things children should know if they are nine, ten, eleven, or twelve years old.

Human reproduction refers to the creation of a new person. After a female develops breasts and pubic hair and begins to menstruate, she can become pregnant if she has sexual intercourse with a developed male who produces sperm. Along with its capacity to become enlarged and harder, the penis, when stimulated, will at times release semen—a whitish, sticky fluid that contains sperm. About the same time a male's testicles begin to produce sperm he is also growing hair around the genitals, showing the first signs of whiskers, and experiencing other physical changes (usually between the ages of eleven and fourteen).

If a sperm unites with the egg cell (called ovum) after sexual intercourse, it is called fertilization. If the fertilized cell attaches to the wall of the uterus, the female becomes pregnant.

Every month one egg matures and travels from one of the ovaries through the Fallopian tube toward the uterus. It can happen that two eggs mature at the same time. Both eggs can be fertilized as the result of sexual intercourse. They then become twins—two males, two females, or one of each. These twins are each in their own amniotic sac. Their genetic makeup is not exactly the same. It is similar, though, since they have the same parents. They are called fraternal twins.

The other kind of twins are called identical twins, and they are always of the same sex. Identical twins are created when a fertilized egg divides in half, and two separate fetuses then begin to develop. Since they came from the same egg and sperm, their genetic makeup is identical and they are in the same amniotic sac. Fraternal twins often look similar, but identical twins are often very hard to tell apart.

The female "period" is called menstruation. The period lasts for about five days each month. This occurs in females who are not pregnant. Blood-enriched tissue is released from the uterine walls through the vagina. So, when a female has a period, she wears a protective sanitary pad or tampon. This is for her comfort and to prevent her clothes from getting stained. Some women feel slightly ill or have cramps just before or during their periods, but most engage in regular activities. Their daily shower or bath should continue during that period so that body odor can be avoided.

The male "wet dream" is called a nocturnal emission. This happens to almost all boys. If not prepared, they think there is something wrong with them. What they have released is semen. It is natural for boys to dream and get excited about sexual thoughts. This causes the penis to get hard or erect. If excited enough, semen comes out. This is called ejaculation. ("Come" or "climax" are other terms used.)

Wet dreams continue for several years. They usually stop when males develop regular opportunities for sexual release, whether through masturbation or sexual intercourse.

Wet dreams are perfectly normal. There is no need to try to control them; they happen to 99 percent of all boys. Without guilt, they can be an enjoyable experience—no matter how strange or sexy the accompanying dreams are. They are only slightly inconvenient, because the bedclothes do get wet and need to be changed. Parents realize this is a sign of a boy's normal growth.

Sometimes boys get erections when sexually excited and sometimes for no apparent reason. Sometimes a small amount of "come" (or "cum") or ejaculate is released. All this is perfectly normal.

MORE ON MASTURBATION

By the time children are ten to twelve years old, masturbation has become an important issue for them. (And, as we mentioned, it's often a big issue for the parents as well.)

Children can simply be told, "Masturbation is a big word for rubbing or stroking the penis, vulva, and/or vagina. It's an enjoyable feeling for both boys and girls. Girls do not ejaculate, but they do lubricate, and at the height of pleasure they have an orgasm. (As with males, "come" or "climax" are other terms used.) No harm can come from doing it. However, like everything else that is pleasant, if it's done more than you really feel like it, it stops being a nice experience. For example, at any given time you may enjoy one ice cream cone, perhaps even two, but the third one makes you feel sick or stuffed. Any good feeling should be treasured and not abused by making it routine or ordinary."

As noted by Mary Calderone, one of the main reasons many adults fail to achieve sexual satisfaction is interference by their parents with the discovery of their bodies as a source of pleasure.

What Children Need to Know: The Adolescent Years

O *ur society often views* adolescence as a disorder or a disease. It's seen as a traumatic period. Yet for many young people adolescence is a wonderful time of life. There are parents today who, when they look back on their earlier years, find that their adolescence was the period when they had the most fun, the most freedom, and the best experiences of love.

We also know that adolescence can be a difficult time for some young people, either during its entire course or for brief, isolated periods. Problems encountered during adolescence, such as a teenager giving birth to a child, would undoubtedly "remap" the teen's life and adversely affect all aspects of the lives of the parents and the child. Quite a few individuals have lifelong troubles that originated in adolescence—delinquency, drug or alcohol abuse, disease, premature parenthood, and a sense of low self-esteem and alienation.

It is significant that young people in the United States are having first intercourse at a younger age. In the '80s, only 20 percent of teen girls had sex by age sixteen and 66 percent by age nineteen. In the mid-'90s, more than 75 percent of adolescents were having intercourse before they graduated from high school. The birth rate for American teenagers in 1995 was 56.8 per thousand, and the pregnancy rate in 1992 was 112 per thousand.

These trends affect a very significant portion of the population. It is easy to say that this can only happen to someone else—to a neighbor's child or to a child from an abusive home. Unfortunately, many parents who think so are deceiving themselves. It is true that lower socioeconomic groups account for a higher percentage of teenage pregnancies, but sexual intercourse among teenagers is a widespread phenomenon now scattered throughout all social and economic classes in this country. Thus, it is vitally important for the parents of today's growing generation to appreciate a few important ideas.

We cannot operate on the assumption that young people are knowledgeable about their own sexuality. Schools that sponsor sexuality education programs often postpone the instruction until after the young person has already begun to experiment with sex. Traditionally, parents themselves have exercised a relatively minimal role in sex education. You may want to review the following questions which, in our experience, are the twenty most frequently asked by teenagers. Consider how you might respond if approached with questions similar to these.

1. How can you tell if you are really in love?
2. Is it all right for people our age [fifteen, sixteen, and seventeen] to have sex?
3. Is masturbation normal?
4. What causes a person to be homosexual? Is it normal?
5. Why is it easier for males to have sex without emotional involvement than for females?
6. How can a girl tell if she has an orgasm?
7. Do pot, alcohol, or other drugs act as a sexual stimulant?
8. Is the pill harmful?
9. How can you tell if you have VD?

10. What is a good contraceptive to use if you are not having sex often?
11. Does the size of one's penis make a difference? How long is the average-size penis?
12. Is it normal if you don't feel ready to have sex?
13. Is it normal to use the mouth in sex play?
14. How come most parents don't tell their children about sex?
15. Can a girl become pregnant the first time she has intercourse?
16. Am I abnormal if I have thoughts about sex with people I know—like in my family?
17. Can I get birth control without my parents knowing about it?
18. How can one avoid pregnancy?
19. How come I get erections even when I'm not thinking about sex?
20. Is porno harmful?

When parents are not askable, young people invariably get their sex information—often misinformation—from their friends. There is a tremendous amount of sex education that occurs without parental awareness or consent in the lunchroom, the locker room, the bathroom, through graffiti, pornography, sex jokes, and the boasts and bravado of some of the presumed sexually active young people.

Young people also receive a great deal of sexual information from movies, TV, ads, rock lyrics, and music videos. Most of it is sensationalistic and distorted. Parents must open the lines of communication and share their own values to help counterbalance the distorted images all around them. Adolescents are aware of the local and national scandals reported almost daily in the press. They sense the hypocrisy when adults establish themselves as models while these same adults are responsible for sexual exploitation in the media. Television uses little restraint in exposing young people to the range of immorality extant in the world. We're not suggesting the imposition of censorship. Instead, we call upon television executives to be aware of the impressionable ages of many of their viewers and act more responsibly, especially in reducing the amount of gratuitous violence that predominates on prime-time network programming and, more recently, on cable. We can't show a scientifically proven causation between TV programming and children's sexual development, but it does appear to us in our clinical work that there is a brutalizing effect in the depiction of excessive violence (often in a sexual context). This is especially true for boys, as expressed in a lack of sensitivity to the feelings of others and a persistent need to dominate. Indeed, this may be a major factor, as children become adults, in the increasing incidence of domestic violence. "Macho" movies are rerun nightly in most markets (in a recent Clint Eastwood film on TV, he was able to drill holes in several men without even getting up from his barber chair). These films were meant for theatrical release, but they end up in our homes on the small screen. In addition, gross humor seems to be getting big ratings, or at least the executives think so. Bathroom humor has reached a new low on the tube. You, too, can express your concerns by writing to networks and shows. Your letters are taken very seriously.

The same networks that feature violence display little sense of responsibility in sexual education. There have been many obstacles for those producers who wished to educate —for instance, not allowing menstruation to be mentioned on *The Waltons,* or prohibiting the use of the term "responsibility" when it referred to contraceptive use on *James at 15.* On the other hand, networks have been very liberal about allowing sex to be used for titillation.

There are sometimes good documentaries and good programs for children, such as *Mr. Rogers* and *Boy Meets World.* Recently, MTV Networks and the Kaiser Family Foundation teamed up to air a series of six public service announcements that examine STDs, HIV, and teen pregnancy while encouraging those who are sexually active to use protection. They also provide a toll-free number to get more information. In the first six months,

150,000 viewers called the hotline, and more than 100,000 of them asked for the booklet. MTV has also had a campaign against teen violence with the help of the Department of Justice and the Department of Education. We applaud MTV and the Kaiser Foundation for their courage and foresight.

Meanwhile, advertisers use sex to peddle their wares. Barely clad women offer tubes of toothpaste, drape themselves over automobiles, and project sales pitches for countless products and services.

Sex is also used to exploit teenagers in their own youth culture. The sexist lyrics of rock music, as well as the Hollywood image of sexiness and success, give ample testimony to this statement.

Society fails to appreciate the high price we pay for allowing the double standard to flourish. Boys are "expected" to have sexual intercourse. If they do not receive this message at home, they certainly get it from their peer group. Girls, on the other hand, are not even expected to be sexual, at least not until they are older or married.

Many families either explicitly or implicitly encourage this double standard. For example, a father will imply that it is okay for his son to have sexual experiences. Often there is a lot of kidding around that gives the impression that if the boy wants to be a man, he is expected to be active sexually. Many parents do communicate to their sons that sex is ideally an expression of love and never a weapon to be used against anyone. We know of many young men who act responsibly and with sensitivity because their parents were able to convey this message clearly and unequivocally. Those young men are less apt to succumb to peer pressure and do not feel a need to prove their masculinity through insincere sexual behavior. Conversely, almost all families, whether or not the parents were sexually active as teenagers, expect their daughters not to engage in sexual activities, or at least expect them to abstain from sexual intercourse until marriage.

This is precisely where the conspiracy begins. Parents mistakenly think their children will use restraint simply because their parents don't want them to engage in sex. Many parents refuse to respond to requests for birth-control information, thinking that if they give such advice their child will see this as permission to engage in sexual behavior. There is risk in everything—but we believe that it is more of a risk *not* to talk to teenagers about their sexuality and birth control.

Parents who are waiting for the "right time" to sex-educate their adolescents may be endangering them more than they realize. Since a significant proportion of teenagers are experimenting with intercourse at fourteen, fifteen, and sixteen, they clearly need concise information before they begin to do so. Research at Johns Hopkins indicates that adolescents are at greatest risk during the first few months of sexual activities. Twenty-two percent of all out-of-wedlock births were found to result from intercourse during the first month after the first act of intercourse; fully 50 percent of all births to unmarried teenagers result from intercourse within the first six months of sexual activity.

The stakes are very high. Research reveals that less than 30 percent of sexually active teenagers use contraception of any form the first time they have sex. Only about 40 percent use some reliable form of contraception as they continue to have sexual relations. All too often we hear the ludicrous complaint made by some extremists that the pill, being the "easiest" form of contraception, is responsible for making girls promiscuous. Actually, use of the pill is unrelated to promiscuity. The sexual irresponsibility of most promiscuous girls is usually the result of ignorance and peer pressure. Many of their parents have not informed them about sex, or have not instilled in them a sense of sexual responsibility. These parents simply establish rules forbidding sex and assume that this is all there is to it.

Establishing rules is sometimes not a deterrent for actions. Teenagers will engage in sexual relations whether we like it or not, and whether they like it or not. We say this quite deliberately. Most teenagers who engage in sexual intercourse don't even enjoy it. The girls virtually never have orgasms the first time they have sexual intercourse. Most boys who have sex as teenagers are more likely to

have an orgasm when they tell their male friends about the experience than when they're actually having sex. Dr. Sylvia Hacker
reported in her research on teenage contraceptive behavior that
young people are indeed engaging in sex more and more and at
younger and younger ages. However, she continues, while the activity is increasing, the comfort with which it is engaged in is not. The
ignorance, guilt, fear, and pressure accompanying the activity are
enormous. It simply defies reality to operate on the assumption that
young people will abstain just because we think they should.

Dr. Thomas Gordon has developed programs that teach parents how to use participatory rule-making. He says, "Denied the
opportunity to participate in establishing a rule, most people feel
imposed upon and resentful...But when people actively participate in setting a rule or making a decision that will affect them,
they are highly motivated to comply with it. Children feel better
about themselves and...they feel they have gained more personal
control over their own lives." Then he gives an example:

Rob, 14 ½, was allowed to buy a dirt bike. One neighbor complained because he drove it in the street, which is against the law.
Another complained that he drove onto their yard, spun his
wheels and dug up their lawn. He also tore up his mom's
flowerbeds. We problem-solved this and came up with several
possible solutions. No bike riding except on camping trips or on
our property. No jumping the bike in flower beds. Mom could
take Rob with his bike to some trails for a couple of hours each
week. He can ride in fields, if he walks the bike there. He can
build a jump on a neighbor's lot. No wheelies on Mom's lawn.
Sell the bike. They threw out some and kept the rest...everyone
happy after two weeks.

This is a simple one—but it illustrates the point, that involving the teens in the decision-making and sharing your concerns
and knowledge with them, brings them into the circle and helps

them to feel part of the solution. (See Recommended Resources for more information on this.)

History has wisely taught us to beware of how myths, fears, and superstitions can influence the political arena. From fear of overstimulating young people or of "putting ideas into their heads that weren't there to begin with," we sometimes deprive them of knowledge that is vital to their well being.

CULTURAL PRESSURES

If parents wish to understand their teenagers and help them through this difficult period in their lives, they would do well to reflect on the cultural and economic climate in which the young people are coming of age. Rapid changes in the social fabric during the post–World War II era have resulted in a confusion of cultural values and a demise of traditional social behavior. We live in a world that puts a premium on achievement and competitiveness. These values may be necessary components of industrial society, but they do cause emotional and psychological stress among adolescents who see them as incompatible with the ideals of love and caring that parents advocate. Society prizes educational achievement and claims that it holds the key to "success," which itself has become a one-dimensional issue of monetary gain. Simultaneously, alternate lifestyles have been downplayed, creating a standardization of behavior that adolescents often feel stifles individual self-expression. All this places an emotional strain on many adolescents.

We all seem to be victims of an age that encourages "instant gratification"—especially reinforced by the styles and fads of the youth culture. Trends among adults contribute equally: the nuclear family, in many instances, no longer provides the required socialization and disciplining functions. The intergenerational conflicts in sexual ethics that result from this breakdown often compound the sense of confusion. It is also vital for parents to perceive that many things have changed since their own teenage years and that values from their own childhood may no longer be dominant social factors.

Today's teenagers face not only changing cultural tides, but bio-logical ones as well. A century ago, the average age of first menstru-ation was seventeen; today it is twelve. The onset of fertility in boys (first ejaculation) has also been decreasing; typically it occurs today between twelve and thirteen years of age. We cannot the ignore the fact that physiologically it is more difficult for today's adolescents to wait until marriage, or until their twenties, to experience sexual intercourse. Today's adolescents not only mature earlier, but delay marriage longer than the teenagers of generations ago.

Understandably, these changing tides have given rise to a new set of legends, such as the popular myth that most teenage females who become pregnant want to have babies, at least on an uncon-scious level. Virtually all research in this field is based on girls who are already pregnant and who decide to give birth. We have studied sexually active but not yet pregnant girls and found that less than 10 percent of teenage girls actually *want* to get pregnant.

In most cases, teenage girls become pregnant because of risk-taking accidents or ignorance. We do not believe that ignorance is the only factor, although it provides a large component of the explanation for pregnancy; for instance, the majority of teenagers don't even know when in their cycle girls are most fertile. We also do not accept the conclusions drawn by some researchers that suggest parents are always at fault. Many parents are askable and do as good a job as possible in relating to their teenage children, yet their children engage in sexual intercourse, and in some cases their daughters or sons are involved in a pregnancy.

Several other myths pervade parents' thinking about their teenagers. It's commonly believed that first intercourse typically occurs in a car, when in fact it most often happens in the parents' home or that of a friend. Parents of a young girl who matures physically before her peers tend to believe that this predisposes her to early sexual relations; actually, there is a relationship between early sexual experiences and growing up in poverty, but not early on the basis of puberty per se. Parents of a teenage boy who shows no interest in dating by age sixteen worry that he may be homosexual (no basis in fact). These and other legends illustrate the dangers of prejudging children based on misinformation.

VULNERABILITY

We need to understand teenage **vulnerability,** an important factor here. Vulnerability occurs not only because of membership in a discriminated-against single-parent family or minority group or because of poverty. There are members of such minority groups who are not vulnerable and who function very well in society. The same holds true for individuals who have been brought up in poverty. Young people feel vulnerable because of poor self-images—they feel they're not pretty, too short, too tall, too developed, or not developed enough. These are bound to be common feelings when the body is manifesting many changes and when peers are developing at many different rates. Young people may also feel there is something wrong with them if their parents are divorced, or if they are adopted. Some adolescents feel vulnerable because they haven't had sex yet, or even because they think it's wrong to feel sexual. Some feel vulnerable because of a physical or mental handicap. Thus, even in the "best" families—families who really care about their children—we can find children who, for a number of reasons, feel vulnerable, and vulnerable teenagers are the *most prone* to engage in irresponsible sexual behavior.

We're clear on what we mean by irresponsible behavior. It is careless, risk-taking sexual activity that could lead, for example, to pregnancy, STD, or psychological trauma. In our judgment, most pregnancies among teenagers are the result of such irresponsible behavior. There are exceptions, but they are few and far between. Put simply, teenagers who feel inferior, inadequate, or insecure—namely, vulnerable—are at greatest risk. Eleanor Roosevelt stated that "no one can make you feel inferior without your consent." We wish that we could impress this message on the hearts of all young people today.

The vulnerability of adolescence is not an indefinite state of affairs. Vulnerable periods can last for days or weeks and crop up at different periods of time. In general, those few young people whose difficulties persist over long periods live in circumstances in which their feelings of powerlessness are constantly reinforced. Statistically, perhaps 70 percent of teens manage quite well without major trauma. Though this fact doesn't minimize the plight of those teens who suffer from STD, pregnancy, emotional difficulties, or drug abuse, it does caution us to proceed with an awareness that we must not treat all adolescents as if they were time bombs waiting to detonate.

In an ironic sense, adolescents suffer some anxiety and uncertainty from all the attention currently being focused on their sexuality. Statistics in the news, magazine articles, and social commentators, though usually well intentioned, have unwittingly helped blow teenage sex out of proportion. It can become both a self-fulfilling prophecy and a source of adolescent grievance. Because the accounts usually concern the perils of teenage sexuality—such as STD and pregnancy—the majority of teens, who are in fact responsible, sometimes resent the idea that they aren't trusted. Interestingly, in a recent study, teenagers stated that sex was not terribly important in their lives. The teens rated "having friendships with members of the same sex," "doing well in school," "having friendships with members of the opposite sex," "being very romantically involved with someone," and "athletics" as more important than "having sex with someone."

We must acknowledge that some young people who engage in sex with love and caring and who use contraceptives are mature. There are sixteen and seventeen year olds who are more mature and capable than some adults. It would be unjust to write this chapter without acknowledging that such adolescents do exist. They are the exceptions, however, and we still feel that teenagers should wait to experience sexual intercourse.

Raising a Child Responsibly in a Sexually Permissive World

COMMUNICATION

If boys and girls openly and freely accept their sexual feelings, they will have questions to ask: Am I ready? What is the best method of birth control for me? If, however, they pretend that they are not sexual, but into idealized, romantic love, or a test of manliness or womanliness, then the important questions don't get asked. Parents who sense that their teenager is or will soon be sexually active have an obligation to bring up the subject of obtaining birth-control information. When your teens ask about sex or birth control, it doesn't mean that they are already sexually active. It is essential that one be sensitive to the child's reason for asking.

In discussions of this nature, it is common for adolescents to put one parent in a dilemma by saying, "I'll tell you, but don't tell Dad (or Mom) about it." The parent's response might be, 'Okay, if that's how you want it, but I wonder if you'd let me use my own judgment here. You are putting me in a difficult situation." If the child insists, then you'll have to go along in order to gain the child's confidence. Once you do make such a promise, keep it *unless* it is a true emergency where you can't risk the consequences of keeping silent.

Parents need to be sensitive to the main worries that young people have. More often than not they are related to being liked or fitting in, making friends, having fun, pursuing interests, and elementary things such as having "enough" spending money. In the sexual areas these worries are translated into an overall concern about being normal. Specifically, they focus on:

- Am I sexually attractive?
- Will I grow more?
- Why do my genitals seem so small or oddly shaped?
- Why am I so slow in developing (pubic hair, breasts, hips, deep voices, whiskers, etc.)?
- Will I ever find someone who will love me?
- Will anyone ever want to have sex with me (or will I ever have the courage to make a sexual overture)?

• Will everyone make fun of me if I admit I want to be a virgin on my wedding night?

Teenagers also have a very strong need for autonomy; this includes wanting parents to respect their differences of opinion. They need **models**, not critics or idols (e.g., from rock music). It is crucial for them to be helpful to others; this enhances their feelings of self-worth and achievement. **Perhaps of greatest benefit is teaching adolescents to accept one another.** Often their first experiences of love and relationships set the tone for future feelings and perceptions of the opposite sex, as well as of themselves.

The double standard makes life extremely difficult for teenagers. Many young girls feel that they won't amount to anything unless some boy wants and loves them (especially if they are disconnected from one or both parents). Most don't realize that almost every boy who impregnates a teenage girl eventually abandons her. Even when teenage parents marry, the family is likely to break up, for one reason or another. It is a rare teenage couple burdened with an unwanted pregnancy that remains intact after five years. We don't want to go into all the details regarding the repercussions of teenage motherhood, but here are a few facts American families should know.

A teenage girl basically has three options when she becomes pregnant. In general, the most traumatic of these options is having the baby, followed closely by giving the child up for adoption. The least residual trauma results from an abortion, though there are important exceptions to this generalization. We play no games on this subject. We clearly and unequivocally believe that if a teenager becomes pregnant, whether due to a mistake, a rape, or a contraceptive failure, she should have the right to choose this third alternative. It is our position that any girl under fifteen is incapable of giving informed consent for sexual intercourse, no matter how sophisticated she may appear. This is legally the case in most states, and the offense is called statutory rape.

Raising a Child Responsibly in a Sexually Permissive World

We respect the views of those who are opposed to abortion; individuals will follow their consciences, but there is general agreement that abortion is not an appropriate form of birth control. In any case, the subject of abortion is not a simple matter, and we work toward eliminating the need for it by promoting realistic and thorough sex education at home and school.

Having stated our position regarding abortion, we would like to review briefly the consequences of a teenager's giving birth. Much poor health and psychological disturbance in our society are related to being born to or being a teenage mother. Frequently the young mother has been smoking, drinking, or using drugs. Low birth weight, infant mortality, physical disabilities, and retardation are common among babies born to teenagers. The chances of such children being physically abused or becoming delinquent or drug-addicted is much greater than if they are born to an older woman. The life script of a teenage mother is also grim. Her chances of finishing school, obtaining a good job, or marrying someone who will be in the picture for more than a few years are minimal. In this context it seems almost trivial to point out that in the next twenty years the American taxpayer will pay in excess of $200 billion (at current prices) for the net results of teenage childbearing. Many of the 500,000 babies born each year to teenagers end up on the welfare rolls.

DECISION-MAKING

It is important for parents to understand the tremendous pressure on teenage girls to have sex. Boys use lines. A study conducted by Planned Parenthood in Chicago surveyed a thousand young men. They were asked if it was okay to lie to a girl, to say that you were in love with her in order to have sex. Seventy percent said yes! Today young people have been softened up by "easy sex" on some of the widely viewed sitcoms, etc. It's hard to imagine how often it occurs in spite of the epidemic of AIDS and teen birth rate.

Many girls are vulnerable to such lines because they don't admit they're having sex at all; they think they're "making love" and acting in a spontaneous and romantic way—and if one is spontaneous and romantic, one doesn't use birth control. To do so would suggest premeditated sex, which they have been taught is wrong. Girls are brainwashed, sometimes by their own parents, not to look upon themselves as sexual human beings. Hence, they give no thought to the possible consequences of their actions, hoping instead that fate will be kind to them.

Ironically, few boys ever have sex spontaneously. They are planning, organizing, and thinking about this for some time. Yet they are not immune to notions of romance or the spontaneity of the moment, nor are they free of ambivalence about their own sexuality. It cannot be too strongly emphasized that young people who know that strong sexual drives are normal and natural can better control their impulses and be more responsible in all areas of sexuality.

It was once thought that a disproportionately high number of pregnancies occurred among black teenage girls because *their* parents loved and wanted more children. This is simply not true. We have worked extensively with black families and have yet to meet parents who wanted their teenage daughter to become pregnant. We seriously doubt that there is more tolerance in one cultural or economic group than another.

It is difficult for most parents to deal with these sensitive issues. The strong sexual drives of their adolescent children may reawaken old fears and anxieties of their own. When we are lecturing to high-school classes, it is not unusual for students to ask, "What you say is all well and good, but what do you do at the peak of passion?" The question is a fair one. It can be countered with: "What are you going to do when you're pregnant?" or "What are you going to do when you get someone pregnant?" One could add, "If you're at the 'peak of passion' and have reached a point of no return, why not consider an alternative to sexual intercourse, such as masturbation? It's satisfying and doesn't create any pregnancies."

To be practical—can there be any significant reduction of irresponsible sexual behavior unless young people feel free to masturbate? When young people say they're horny, they mean it. They feel sexual tension. They want relief. In our judgment, the best relief for sexual excitement and tension for teenagers is masturbation.

Teenagers involved in an intimate relationship often find that in the midst of kissing and heavy petting, sexual tensions become very compelling. At those times it's nearly impossible to wait until they get home to masturbate. Sometimes adolescents are not able to delay the impulse toward sexual release, and unfortunately this often leads to unplanned sexual intercourse. In these situations, mutual masturbation may be a realistic alternative. There is a risk in this, as it may progress to intercourse, but there is an even greater risk among those couples who move immediately to intercourse.

Sometimes we have been accused of giving contradictory messages. For instance, we state very clearly that we think sexual intercourse is good—yet we don't want teenagers to engage in it. (Here we are not referring to other forms of sexual expression in caring relationships, such as kissing, necking, or mutual masturbation.) We think that young people should wait until they are *at least* eighteen and off to college, working or living on their own, to have sexual intercourse. A person in his or her later teen years knows more, is more mature, and can deal better with the consequences of even irresponsible behaviors. We see no contradiction here. One must reach a certain age to vote, drive a car, or sign a contract. There are good moral and health reasons for parents to urge their children to abstain while they are still at home. After a child is employed or off to college, we can only hope (and pray) that our moral influence remains a vital force in their lives. By having the discussion early, you are giving children the opportunity to think before they act.

There are many types and degrees of sexual behavior. Some people are more sexual with each other when they hold hands or look into each other's eyes than when engaging in actual intercourse. There can be more sexual excitement in kissing or caressing than in coitus. Much of what constitutes sexual intercourse is not even enjoyable for many young people because they don't have enough understanding of how to enjoy each other and to appreciate its deeper meaning. Often the motivation to have sexual relations is for a false notion of self-respect rather than pleasure or intimacy. For boys, sex often means proving masculinity—for girls, desirability or femininity. As suggested by Gisela Konopka, "In our culture, success for a girl means being attractive and acceptable to boys."

There is a great deal of pressure put on adolescents to engage in sexual relations. Many we know who have "gone all the way" are among the most bored, alienated, and unhappy young people, who drift from one sexual partner to another without getting to know one another. Sex without intimacy is rarely a satisfying experience. Brief encounters can be psychologically damaging to young people. That's why it's so important to start sexuality education early!

It is sometimes tempting to believe that the pendulum is swinging back to more traditional ways of thinking. For instance, a recent Educational Communications (Lake Forest, Illinois) survey of top high-school students (those listed in *Who's Who among American High School Students*) reported that they were predominantly responsible and conservative in their sexual attitudes. Seventy-six percent said they had not had sexual intercourse, and only 8 percent said they favored couples living together before marriage. Such elitist groups do tend to be more knowledgeable about sex, and they are generally less vulnerable than the average student. The study substantiates our view that some informed adolescents delay their first sexual intercourse until after high school.

Recent studies reveal that about 90% of college students—at least in the nonsectarian universities—will have had sexual intercourse before they graduate.

BETWEEN PARENTS AND CHILDREN

The most important message we have for parents is this: **Let your children know that no matter what they do, you will never reject them.**

Raising a Child Responsibly in a Sexually Permissive World

The most responsible message you can give is, "You are our child; no matter what happens, you can come to us and we'll help you."

Some of you may remember the furor created in 1975 when former First Lady Betty Ford said, "I do not believe in premarital relationships, but I realize that many in today's generation do not share my views. However, this must never cause us to withdraw the love, the counseling and the understanding that they may need now more than ever before." She created a media sensation when she acknowledged the possibility that her daughter might choose to have premarital sex. When her view was more soberly reviewed, the vast majority of the American public appreciated what she had said. Most ministers endorsed her positions. This was a good example of media overreaction; they created the impression that Mrs. Ford's statement was permissive and somehow dangerous.

We appreciate the openness and honesty of Betty Ford's statement. There was clearly a sense of caring and respect between parent and child. Children who are allowed to work out their own values find generally that it is the parents' important values they select in the end. Parents who take an uncompromisingly harsh position devoid of mutual trust are inviting tragedy. Nearly a million teenagers run away from home each year in this country. Girls account for almost half this number; as many as 40 percent of them run away because they are pregnant. Fear is a prime factor as evidenced in these statements: "My father said that if I ever became pregnant he'd kill me"; "My mother said that if I ever became pregnant I shouldn't come home." These runaways face horrors on the streets. Many end up the victims of pimps who immediately turn them into prostitutes. Pregnancy is also a significant reason for suicide among teenage girls.

Even parents who have good relationships with their offspring can reach an impasse when it comes to speaking openly and freely about sexuality. Sometimes one can grasp a good opportunity—an article in the newspaper, a "Dear Abby" column, or a television show where a couple has sex on the first date (!)— and make this into a teachable moment. Don't get discouraged if your child is silent—they are no doubt listening. Some times it works to leave a well-illustrated sexuality education book in a not-too-conspicuous place. (See Recommended Books.) The child will no doubt become curious.

Teenagers are entitled to privacy. They should not be expected to tell parents everything. This can be painful to caring parents who feel they can be of little help if their teenagers don't reveal the intimacies and intricacies of their lives. Sometimes teenagers kid around to mask their real feelings or say what they assume the parents want to hear.

Sometimes parents who genuinely mean well stumble in the beginning. Here is a list of phrases guaranteed to turn off young people:

- I want to have a serious talk with you.
- We trust you.
- When I was your age...
- Because we say so.
- As long as I don't know about it.
- Act your age.
- It's about time you...(got good grades, cleaned your room).
- Just a minute.
- Ask your father/mother.
- Are you telling me the truth?
- That's not your idea, is it?
- Don't you dare to talk to me that way.
- Get off your high horse.
- Wipe that smile off your face.
- What will the neighbors say?
- After all we've done for you...
- I told you so!

Parents need to be especially careful when teens say they're in love. If you respond with "You'll get over it," "When you get older you'll laugh about it," or "It's puppy love," you're likely to push them away. Take it seriously; it might be helpful to read the section for teenagers on how to tell when you are in love. It could help you and your child make distinctions between mature and immature love.

It is not easy to give advice about what to do if children want to date before you think they're ready. You can validate their feelings even as you refuse their demands. Hold to your principles—and don't allow them to sway you with comments that you are old-fashioned or that all the other kids in the neighborhood have more permissive parents. Acknowledge that you may be different (or old-fashioned, or too strict, etc.) from others, but don't get caught debating your own parental qualifications.

There are, however, many situations in the lives of teenagers that are not subject to parental control. The following incident actually happened to an acquaintance of ours. A seventeen-year-old girl called her mother late at night and told her that she and her boyfriend had been drinking quite a bit. It was too late for her to get public transportation, and the boyfriend offered to take her home on his motorcycle. Our friend did not drive and in her anxiety could not think of an alternative solution such as a taxi. She responded by telling the daughter to stay overnight; she admitted later that she preferred to have her daughter risk pregnancy than risking an accident. We all must use common sense in some situations, even when it violates our principles.

While we have stressed the importance of knowledge throughout this book, we want to affirm that it is no guarantee of intelligent behavior. Most people have read the Surgeon General's warning about the smoking of cigarettes and the risk of lung cancer, yet many intelligent people do smoke. Now we know that our teens are aware that tobacco companies have been targeting young people. Resisting these huge forces is not easy—any more than it's easy to resist the seductive commercial invitations to sexuality. In the same vein, decisions about sex are not necessarily tied to knowledge. (See Chapter Two.) Even knowledgeable adults sometimes engage in irresponsible sexual behavior. We still insist that with knowledge there is generally more responsible behavior than without it—but knowledge by itself is not sufficient.

Feelings and levels of emotional maturity often are more important than knowledge. Providing information per se is not the main point in being an askable parent; one must also be able to identify with children and their feelings. Teenagers in general express a wide range of emotions. "I don't feel good about myself and won't until I have a boyfriend [girlfriend]." "I'm mortified because everyone is having sex and I'm the only one who isn't." We sometimes forget that we need to **support** young people who **don't** want to have sex.

We suggest providing guidelines for your children rather than rigid rules, which are often broken, either secretly or defiantly. How many families, believe, for example, that if a teenager is home before midnight no sexual activity can take place? Do families understand, as do teenagers, that one certainly can have sex before midnight as well as after this arbitrary hour? It might be useful to talk over such an issues with your son or daughter. Make it clear that your main concern in having your child home at a reasonable hour is your worry about the possibility of muggings, robberies, or accidents as a result of drunken driving, all of which do occur more frequently after midnight. Explain that you simply have a hang-up—you can sleep better knowing your child is safe at home. Children will be more responsive to their parents' needs if they are part of the discussion on rules ahead of time.

Many parents are confronted with the dilemma of having a teenager return home from college with a lover and want to sleep with the lover during the visit. Many parents accept the situation, but those who disapprove must examine the consequences of their various responses. To threaten to do something extreme, such as cutting off college tuition, could result in a complete severance of family ties. If you are uncomfortable with the idea because of younger children, or for moral or religious reasons, it is naturally your right to forbid sharing a bed in your home. Before making your decision, however, you may wish to consider things from the young people's perspective. "We're sleeping together at school," they reason, "so why pretend at home that the situation doesn't exist?" If that sensible question sometimes seems defiant, it is probably because behind it lies an honest plea for parental acceptance of their sexuality. We believe that, in most cases, granting that acceptance can only improve family relationships.

There is no evidence that living together sets the stage for unhappy marriages or divorce. If our own son came home and announced he wanted to marry a girl on relatively short acquaintance, we can imagine ourselves saying, "Why don't you live together first and get to know each other?" In any event, it is best to balance your own beliefs with an open responsiveness to your child's choice, rather than worrying about neighbors, relatives, or anyone else.

Parents must also realize that it is natural for teens to take risks and make mistakes. Adolescence is a time for testing relationships and personal abilities. Teenagers test reactions to their behavior and try to decide on personal interests and goals, balancing them with the opportunities they perceive in society. The situation is critical only when they don't learn from these trials and errors along the way.

In Hermann Hesse's *Siddhartha*, an important book in our adolescence, the hero observes: "Knowledge can be communicated, but not wisdom." Ultimately, as parents and a society, we need to give teens more support for their own stated priorities, dreams, and ambitions. While we are doing this, we can empathize with young people and say we understand the pressures to engage in sexual intercourse—pressures that often push them away from their dreams. But at the same time we might say, "All right. We know that you are under pressures, that rock music lyrics and videos encourage you to have sex, but let me ask you: When you get pregnant, are you going to get a letter of congratulations from your favorite rock star? When you need an abortion, are the *Baywatch* writers going to send you the money?"

We have to let these young people know that their mothers aren't going to take care of their babies: "You've got a lot of nerve! Your poor mother? Why should she take care of your baby? That's not fair."

LETTERS FROM TEENAGERS

We receive a lot of letters from adolescents who have read one of our books or attended a lecture. They often pose problems or describe how hard it is to maintain the integrity of their beliefs. Here are some of their own words:

Dear Dr. Sol Gordon,

I read your book, "You Would If You Loved Me," and really enjoyed it…me and all my friends, we've all been through breaking up because we wouldn't give him the main thing he wanted. Our hearts were all, of course, broken, and we even regretted (a little) not doing that, but we all know it was for the better.

Me and my boyfriend were together for 10 months and broke up for (mostly) that reason (sex!?). I always told him near the beginning of our relationship that he had better break up with me if he wanted to do that, but he'd always tell me that that wasn't what he wanted. He always wanted a fun relationship, so we just kept on going!!

During the relationship he'd always try to pressure me in doing that, but I would always have excuses, or get mad at him, or remind him of the things that we had talked about earlier. Some of my excuses were: that I had my period; I had to be home at 12:00, and if I was late dad would kill both of us; that none of my other friends had done it and I didn't want to be the first one; and also just plainly say "no"!!! He'd of course get mad at me but it was mostly his fault that I would have to leave him in that state of "hard-on."

I would always try to tell him that we could have fun with each other and not have to do that. Because it's true: "If you really care for me and love me and love this relationship then you shouldn't pressure me, because none of this would be worth it or just be wasted if we had to break up for this dumb reason!!" So, I guess we did break up, and we are (kind of) good friends now. But from what I've heard, he still hasn't done that yet so he might just give up!

Mr. Gordon,

A couple of weeks ago two guys invited my girlfriend and I to a party. The whole night this one guy kept trying to get me to have sex with him, so I thought I'd write and tell you his lines. First of all, he kept trying to get me high all night, constantly lifting a beer to my lips and offering me a joint to smoke; he was trying to get me so high that I couldn't say "no." Then he started asking me if I wanted to go back to his place (he was three years older than me.)

He kept trying to kiss me and put his hands on my boobs, and I finally just told him "no sex." The last thing I remember of that terrible evening was that he said even though I didn't let him do anything that I was the nicest girl he'd ever been with. I wondered how many other girls he'd said that to! I was afraid he was going to rape me, and I finally got away by faking being sick from all the beer. Why are some guys so pushy they're willing to practically sit on top of you to get what they want?

Mr. Gordon,

I'm a 13-year-old girl, and my problem is this really cute guy who goes to my school. I fell in love with him, and one night we really started making out at his parents' place. Since then we have done **everything** but go all the way. We'll both be naked, and he will **beg** and **beg** me to go all the way. I'm too young to get pregnant and I don't know how to use any type of birth control. I want to be the one responsible for it. Also, we have to sneak and hide, which you said in your book was a no-no. Once my dad found out I had been over there, and he called me a slut, whore, etc. And he doesn't even know what happened. I really hate sneaking around, and my dad will throw me out if he finds out. Is it a line when you tell the guy "no" and he cries?

Dear Sir:
I am a 15-year-old male from Michigan, and I have just finished reading your "lines" book, *You Would If You Loved Me*.[1]
I had no idea that guys were only after sex or were so lustful.
It surprised me that it was the guys' fault for the 1,000,000
adolescent pregnancies. I think that more emphasis should be
placed on the word "no". Every girl should know this. I have
always thought that there's no excuse for getting a girl pregnant, but it seems like you are trying to lay a guilt trip on the
males of the world. I'm not saying that it's the girl's fault
either. The responsibility should be a mutually shared and
wanted satisfying adventure. I can't understand it being anything else.

Dear Dr. Gordon:
Could you give me some advice? I am a junior in high school
here in New York, and I am a Christian. I have very funda-
mentalist values toward the subject of sex and feel that people
should wait until marriage. I believe God wants it that way.
But that's my opinion.

I am now dating a young Christian man who I really love.
We've discussed sex, and we're both virgins. A couple of days
ago he told me that he wants to make love to me and wants to
wait for the right time. Dr. Gordon, I'm having trouble trying
to remain in my virgin status. I would like to make love. What
if it hurt our relationship or I don't marry him eventually? I
want to be a virgin for my husband—what if I get hurt? Birth
control is not the problem—the problem for me is a matter of
religious values. Please help! I care enough for him to give up
my virginity, but I still have these doubts.

---

1. A new edition is retitled, *Seduction Lines Heard 'Round the World.*

Dear Dr. Sol,

...Well, to get to the real problem, I'm a sophomore in high school, and I have a hang-up about sex. Not your average teenage "oh isn't he a hunk." At dances and other places when I see a boy I like I go after him, and I really have had a lot of sexual relations. I have a terrible reputation. But I consider myself to be fairly intelligent—I just can't help it. I don't have any friends, except for these guys that come to see me for "favors." I tell myself to stop doing it, but I can't seem to—it's compulsory. My parents don't know anything about it, so please don't tell them I'm this way. But they're beginning to suspect. Please help me!

P.S. I hope you don't think this is a joke.

In concluding the chapter, we'd like to summarize our main messages to young people.

1. Girls get pregnant because they have sexual intercourse.
2. Regardless of what the movies and the music tell you, it's not romantic to have sex without birth control, it's stupid.
3. When someone says, "If you really love me, you'll have sex with me," it's *always* a line.
4. Sex is never a test or proof of love.
5. Sex is never a test or proof of masculinity or femininity.
6. More than 85 percent of all boys who impregnate teenage girls will eventually abandon them.
7. Girls who feel they don't amount to anything unless some boy loves them should realize that self-worth never comes from someone else.
8. People who feel good about themselves tend to be more responsible about their sexual behavior.
9. Of the ten most important things in a relationship, sex is number nine. Number one is love and caring.
10. The best test of a relationship is to see what happens when you hold off having sexual intercourse.

CHAPTER NINE

Parents' Questions about Adolescence

I t is during their children's adolescence that many parents
have the most difficulty understanding, and responding to,
sexual issues. Living with adolescents revives memories parents retain of their own teenage years, so they relive some of those
feelings. Fears, joys, and pains are jolted from musty memory
banks and sometimes distort the present.

DISCIPLINE AND RULES

A matter of critical importance for many families is how to handle authentic differences of opinion between the parents about
management of their child. This is especially important in the
area of sexuality because the consequences could be serious.
Differences between parents can range from when to allow a child
to go out on a date, to an appropriate curfew time, to attitudes on
how to handle male and female children. These differences may
generate real conflicts, e.g., "You're too hard on the children" or
"You don't trust the children enough." This can have serious consequences for the marital relationship, and also children may
exploit the differences for their own benefit.

Raising a Child Responsibly in a Sexually Permissive World

It is imperative that parents work through these conflicts and present a unified front. Sometimes one can take a flexible approach and say, "Listen…your father [mother] and I disagree, but for now we're going to go with my point of view. If that doesn't work, in six months we'll consider another alternative." Not all families are open to this kind of compromise, and parents may prefer to negotiate privately without informing the child of the process involved. Sometimes it's even worth doing a little research in the library; we're not suggesting that experts know it all, but sometimes you can get some good ideas that apply to your own situation. In some families it's even possible to have a family conference at which grievances are aired and solutions shared, or a community conference where families share their feelings about rules and limits. Allowing young people to negotiate within predetermined limits can foster excellent self-esteem and be a helpful preparation for adult life.

The risk to the children is less serious when parents agree on their approach (permissive, authoritarian, or democratic) than when they involve the children in parental battles of will. Even joking remarks such as "That's the way women are" or "All men are the same" can be harmful. Be aware that conflicts over a child can camouflage conflicts that really exist in the marriage. In these situations, parents "choose" to fight over a child rather than face the difficulties that exist between themselves.

Here are some parents' questions on discipline and rules and our answers to them.

• *I'm a father whose fifteen-year-old son demands to know why I keep trying to influence him by setting rules for his behavior when, he argues, he's "grown-up." I'm not really sure how to answer him, and this has become a real conflict between us.*
You've raised a good question, and we're sure that parents of twelve and thirteen year olds have heard similar arguments from their children. Parents sometimes intuitively know that they need

to enforce discipline within the family, but are stymied when asked their rationale for doing so.

Parents can tell their children, "It's important to us that you become a healthy, happy adult. That's why we say no alcohol or drugs, because these things interfere with physical and psychological development. We want you home at night by a reasonable time so that you can get the sleep you need and we know you're not in danger. We also say no sexual intercourse, because it's too much of a risk. We feel that as long as you still live with us it's our responsibility to help you, to protect you."

• *I'm the mother of a sixteen-year-old son, and I feel that in the area of sex my son is particularly vulnerable and may be getting himself into some trouble. How can I express my concern for him without revealing the mistakes I feel I've made in my own life in the past?*

Even conservative parents reach adulthood with the feeling that they have made some mistakes in past relationships and sexual behavior. They fear, on the one hand, being untruthful if they fail to divulge these experiences to children, and, on the other hand, being labeled hypocritical when they tell children to "do as I say, not as I did."

In this situation, a balance is important. It's not advisable to share the intimate details of your sexual life, good or bad. Acknowledging is not an open invitation to be specific about the details. This raises the question of how specific to get in setting sexually related standards for children. A conservative parent and colleague of ours, Alison Deming, surprised herself immensely when she told her son, "Don't ever knowingly use your penis as a weapon to hurt somebody." After she recovered from her shock at being so candid with her son, she found that the resulting conversation was one of the most rewarding ever. Somehow or other, girls are told that they need to protect themselves, but we neglect to give similar messages to boys.

Some parents, especially fathers, go so far as to imply that there might be something wrong with the teenage son who is still a virgin at sixteen or seventeen. This message is often conveyed in jokes and bawdy stories about "what hell-raisers we were when we were growing up." Boys benefit from information regarding self-control, discipline, and responsibility just as much as girls do.

• *What is your position on parental notification in cases where minor children seek prescription contraceptives or other medical services?*
It is natural and desirable for parents to know about important events and developments in their children's lives. Ideally, this occurs in the context of loving parent–child relationships in which important issues are open for discussion. There are, however, many families in which such communication does not take place. The question arises: in instances where teenagers obtain birth-control help from clinics, is it justifiable or desirable for the clinic to notify the parents, with or without the minor's consent?

We believe that the health and welfare of the child must take precedence over other considerations. A survey of young patients at federally funded family-planning clinics suggested that 25 percent of these patients would stop applying for prescription contraceptives if their parents were notified. Only 2 percent said they would stop sexual activity as the result. In another study, 58 percent of sexually experienced teens report not using contraception every time they have intercourse. Thirty-six percent of those who have had intercourse say they never talked with their partner about preventing pregnancy; 40 percent never talked with the partner about preventing STDs.

No contraceptive method affects a teenager's health more adversely than pregnancy; teenagers are five times more likely to die from pregnancy-related causes than from use of the pill.

Rabbi Marvin Schwab (Temple Ohr Rishon-Sunrise) put it very well in the *Sacramento Bee*, Jan. 2, 1999, in response to a question from the Religion Editor: "Given the dangers of unpro-tected sex, actress Sharon Stone says that if you truly love your children, you need to supply condoms in your home and do it nonjudgmentally. Do you agree?"

The first issue here is the context, and the context of Sharon Stone's statement is one of saving lives. The danger of HIV infection is very real, and it leads to a fatal disease. In Jewish law, all the precepts of Judaism except three (the prohibitions against committing murder, incest and idolatry in public) may be transgressed in order to save a life. Therefore, if mak-ing condoms accessible means that unprotected (and there-fore risky) sex will be prevented, then the condoms should be made available. Does this mean that promiscuity is approved? No. Does this mean that 10-year-olds should be having sex? No. Does this mean that the condoms should appear without any discussion of sexual morality between parents and chil-dren? No. It means just the opposite of all of these, and it means saving the lives of our children is the most important ideal we can hold dear.

Congress cannot legislate either family solidarity or responsi-ble behavior. We believe that adolescents must be allowed to pro-tect their health whether or not they choose to listen to good counsel. We must also remember that today's teenagers didn't cre-ate the "sexual revolution"—they are its victims.

PHYSICAL MATTERS

• *My daughter approached me with a question recently, and I'm not sure I handled it very well. She had been reading a book on sexuality addressed to young teens and was especially concerned about first intercourse and the role of the hymen. She has always been athletic and was worried that her hymen might have rup-tured in vigorous exercise. I wasn't sure how to describe the hymen or how to find it, and I'm wondering if there was some underlying message in her question.*

Your question highlights the serious concerns which young teenagers have in relation to sexual intercourse and the various aspects of sexual expression. The hymen is no longer prized as a symbol of virtue (although for some couples the bride's virginity is significant to their marriage).

As your daughter suspected, exercise can break the hymen so that it is no longer there at first intercourse. Some females are born with a small or undetectable hymen, while in others it is pronounced. Through the use of tampons or through masturbation the hymen is sometimes broken.

Women who reach first intercourse with an intact hymen are sometimes concerned about painful penetration of the penis. Great gentleness on the part of the male is urged, along with some lubrication. Some bleeding may occur, and this is perfectly normal. Because of these circumstances and general inexperience, first sexual intercourse is not very enjoyable for many people.

You might tell your daughter that it's unwise for her to engage in sexual intercourse while still a teenager. As an adult, she'll be better able to make her own decisions concerning premarital sexual experiences. The important aspect here is not the hymen itself, but rather the love and caring between herself and her future partner and the compatibility of their values and goals.

This question also gives us an opportunity to address other fears that both boys and girls have about first sexual experiences. Boys worry whether they will be able to find the girl's vagina, whether they will be able to penetrate, and whether their penis will remain erect. Girls worry that they may appear clumsy or will not have an orgasm. These "performance" anxieties again focus mistakenly on the mechanics of sex rather than on the partners' feelings and the meaningful aspects of the relationship. In today's culture, unless your children live in an isolation booth, they will be sexually stimulated, aware, and full of questions.

Parents can help their children sort through these feelings to anticipate sexual intercourse as adults and in the process come to a better understanding of themselves, other people, and the nature of sexuality in general. While a girl of your daughter's age should not be **sexually active,** it is good for her to be *intellectually and emotionally* prepared so that sex and intimate relationships are not painful surprises later on.

• *In this age of conformity, popularity, and good looks, how do parents comfort children who don't feel themselves to be sexually attractive, let alone accepted by a peer group? We have a daughter who is fourteen years old, is small for her age, and has a severe case of acne. She is so troubled by her feelings of inferiority, especially in relation to boys, that even her ordinarily good grades are beginning to suffer.*
We're sure we'd look foolish if we tried to offer a simple answer to this question. Cliques and exclusive friendship groups dominate at this age. It is also a time when children can be cruel to one another. Sometimes the best thing is to help your child sweat it out and increase activities with the family that increase self-esteem, while decreasing exposure to sarcastic and cynical entertainment. It's good to take a stand and say you find such entertainment demeaning. This applies to many situations in which children are not popular for one reason or another: the handicapped (see also Chapter 12), the unattractive, and those who appear to possess characteristics of the opposite sex.

You can help your child have a good relationship with you, her parents. Don't lie or gloss over as in, "If only you would try harder, everything would be all right," or "The only thing that counts is a good personality." Empathize with the child, suggesting that you know how difficult it is, but that you also know that as she gets older her intellectual and personality development will in fact become more important than her appearance, which will also change. She may not believe it, but you have to.

MASTURBATION

• *I'm a forty-two-year-old mother whose son is now fourteen. Often when I knock on his door, it takes him a long time to answer, and he occasionally spends a lot of time in the bathroom. I'm sure he's masturbating a lot, and despite all I've read about masturbation being "healthy" I can't seem to shake the feeling that it's wrong. Should I talk with my son about this?*

This sounds more like a personal dilemma rather than a specific conflict or problem between yourself and your son. What you say is true—it is difficult to overcome the childhood conditioning that masturbation is bad or to be feared. We appreciate your courage and openness and would like to make some comments you might find helpful.

Adolescents can be helped to appreciate that masturbation is a healthy, normal way of expressing and enjoying their sexual feelings and relieving sexual tensions. Furthermore, why shouldn't adults be able to masturbate comfortably and pleasurably when opportunities for sex with their partners are not available?

Society pays a big price for its repressive views on masturbation. Clinical data and research on persons who have committed violent sexual crimes strongly suggests a relationship between feelings of guilt and punishment for childhood masturbation and the need to dominate or violate women or children. These symptoms also seem to go along with early parental rejection or deprivation.

Society has so brainwashed young men that many feel it's unmanly to masturbate once they've experienced sexual intercourse. Consequently, our country has left a sad reservoir of unwanted children in such places as Japan, Vietnam, and Thailand. To many men, prostitution, or even rape, seem preferable to masturbation. This is no small matter.

Two brief anecdotes will illuminate the ways in which misperceptions continue to inhabit people's attitudes:

An editor of a medical journal asked us to respond to a question posed by a seventeen-year-old boy who stated that he couldn't speak to a female or go to a dance without getting an erection. The young man had pleaded for help. He especially asked that no one make fun of him; it was a serious matter for him. He also didn't want to be told that he'd get over it (which, the editor revealed, was the answer several experts offered nonetheless). We suggested to the young man that he simply masturbate before he went to a dance or had a date. If he felt it was necessary, he could repeat the process during the course of the evening. He should then be able to enjoy a relaxed night out without embarrassment. The editor refused to print our reply, claiming that it was not "professional" advice; we, however, still can't think of a better solution. The unpredictability of erections can be a great source of anxiety for young men. With masturbation, a boy can gain a reassuring sense of self-mastery and control.

Ten years ago one of us spoke before the mental-health association in an upstate New York community. Reference was made to masturbation. A reporter present accurately recorded what had been said. When the article was submitted to the editor, he refused to use the word "masturbation," since he felt that this was inappropriate terminology for a "family" newspaper. A debate then ensued among the staff members regarding a proper substitute for the word. Two were considered: "self-abuse" and "self-pleasuring." It was to the staff's credit that they finally agreed to use "self-pleasuring."

The treatment of choice for preorgasmic women involves learning how to enjoy self-pleasuring. Often women who have been preorgasmic for many years achieve their first orgasms through masturbation and then go on to become orgasmic with their partners as well.

For some people with sexual problems, masturbation can be a therapeutic tool where psychotherapy alone has failed. Men who suffer from premature ejaculation or impotence often learn greater control by using masturbation. In the last few decades, attitudes concerning masturbation have done a dramatic about-face among professionals, and these enlightened views are gradually filtering into the population at large.

Sure, we've come a long way. Woody Allen stated in one of his films that he enjoys masturbation—at least he's having sex with someone he loves. Some religious groups still frown upon it, yet even the most extreme opponents in the Catholic Church, for example, have modified their position considerably during the last thirty years. The book *Sexual Morality: A Catholic Perspective*, by the conservative theologian Philip S. Keane, provides ample testimony to this fact. We predict that twenty years from now no one will give masturbation another thought, except to acknowledge its pleasurable aspects.

Regardless of such idealistic prophecies, some parents will remain uncomfortable with masturbation, but the chain of anxiety can be broken by teaching your children to understand and accept their sexual impulses. Parents may not like to use words such as "masturbation" or expressions such as "playing with yourself." We're indebted to our colleague Gloria Blum for the concept of "private touching." It rightly suggests that masturbating, like other forms of sexuality, is not a public matter.

Our overall position is as follows: There is no evidence that all healthy people masturbate or that you must masturbate to be healthy. Once may be too much if you don't enjoy it. There are people—especially some adult women—who have no memory of ever masturbating and who suffer no apparent ill effects. Some mature men and women give up masturbation entirely after they obtain regular opportunities for sexual intercourse; others enjoy masturbation more than coital sex. Most people continue to masturbate at some time or other throughout their entire lives.

In effect, we're suggesting that your concern about your child's "problem" is more than likely an indication of your own inhibitions. Masturbation should be a concern only when it is compulsively performed, and then it is a symptom of some other difficulty—in the same way that overindulgence in food and alcohol are symptoms of anxiety in other areas of a person's life. (People don't get drunk because they are thirsty.)

It is the responsibility of the parent to make sure that children understand that masturbation in private is normal. Beyond that, the parent should make judgments as to whether or not the child is experiencing difficulties. Ask yourself if your child (1) has friends, (2) enjoys life, and (3) treats people with respect (is neither constantly rebellious nor overcompliant).

DATING

• *My fifteen-year-old daughter announced that she was going on a date with a boy she met that afternoon. (My daughter said she was going to go with him whether I liked it or not, and she's been in such a depressed, angry mood lately that I'm sure she would disobey me if I forbade it.)*

Let us tell an actual story of what one parent did in response to this situation. When Mrs. Jones realized that her daughter was going to go out with this young man no matter what she said, she said yes but with one commitment: the boy must come to the house and pick the girl up personally. When he arrived, Mrs. Jones invited him into the kitchen privately, saying, "I'd like to talk to you for a minute." She asked to see his driver's license. She then copied down the name, address, and license number and said, "You seem like a fine young man, but I think you can understand why I have reservations about my daughter, who is much younger, going out with you" (the young man was eighteen). "She is determined, so I want you to know that if she isn't home by eleven o'clock I will call the police immediately. Enjoy and have a good time." When the daughter returned at ten-thirty, the mother asked if she had had a good time and she answered, "Not really. From about nine-thirty on, he kept asking what time it was. I guess you were right; I didn't like him that much anyway." And that was that.

The whole issue of dating is a very complicated one. It's easy enough for us to state what seems appropriate, but obviously the follow-through is much more difficult. Children test us from time to time. Teens often think *their* parents are the most conservative, old-fashioned, meanest that exist. Virtually all parents face this dilemma, particularly in a world where children and adults are bombarded by sexual stimulation everywhere they look. "Get them young" seems to be the plan (certainly the tobacco industry has discovered the rewards in this approach). Caring parents have a responsibility to establish rules, within which teens can make choices.

Chaperones are a minimal necessity for parties that include anyone under eighteen. Group dates rather than individual dates are preferred for young teenagers. This is often a great relief to the young people themselves. Though peer pressure seems to encourage individual dating, young people themselves want the security of other people present.

Curfews need to be established, with an absolutely clear statement that no matter what happens, the child must call if there's some reason for a late homecoming. The very best thing is for parents to establish contacts with one another, such as a simple telephone call saying, "My son is going to take out your daughter [or my daughter is going out with your son]. I just wanted you to know my telephone number."

"Don't you trust me?" is a difficult question most adolescents constantly pose. A simple response is, "Of course we do, but we still have to take precautions that represent your best interests, whether they seem rational to you or not and whether you like it or not." Another typical complaint is, "Oh, Mom/Dad, you're treating me like a baby." The best response is, "I'm sorry it feels that way to you, but I still have to use my best judgment. That's what families are all about. We all have rules to abide by—at home, at school, and at work." If you have been using family meetings all along to decide the "rules of the house" and to share concerns and plans and joys, this stage will be much easier.

All parents worry that their children might engage in sexual intercourse when they are too young. They rightly want to protect the child from rash mistakes, such as pregnancy, sexually transmitted disease, and the psychological problems related to premature sexual encounters. Both boys and girls are at risk here, though girls suffer more. There are three main reasons: (1) the girl is the only one who gets pregnant; (2) girls are often asymptomatic with respect to some STDs (the boy usually knows he has it); and (3) in our "sexist" society, the girl often has sex because of the possibility of love, but the boy usually has sex because of the likelihood of sex—no small matter, however much we favor responsible behavior for both sexes. Both boys and girls are the victims of ad campaigns—in commercials and in the shows that encourage these attitudes.

You can talk to children about sexuality without giving them the impression you are proposing that they have sex. Here is a true story. A twelve-year-old girl asked her mother whether or not it was possible to become pregnant without being married. The mother, fearful of giving the girl "ideas," answered that it was not possible to get pregnant unless one had in fact gotten married. When this woman's older daughter learned of the answer her mother had given, she insisted that the mother talk to the girl again. The mother reluctantly did and discovered to her horror that her little twelve-year-old daughter had been having intercourse with the boy down the street and was really inquiring whether or not she could get pregnant from these experiences. The mother, in believing that talking about sex equaled giving permission, barely escaped a family tragedy.

The risk related to talking about sex and birth control with teenagers is far less than the risk associated with not talking about it. It's astonishing how many girls get pregnant because they have accepted what appears to be the parental message: If you talk or think about it, you'll do it; if you prepare for sex or you premeditate it, there's something wrong with you. The mass media only reinforce the message: "How romantic it is to just let it happen." Birth control is conspicuously absent from movies, television, and romance novels. Let's face it: the CEOs really don't have our children's best interests in mind. These matters are discussed in the better young-adult books, such as those by Judy Blume and Gloria D. Miklowitz, which provide an opportunity for some rehearsal on the adolescent's part.

• *My twelve-year-old daughter wants to go to a boy–girl party, and I'm not convinced there are going to be any adults present.* Our response is not to let her go unless you feel certain chaperones will be there. Insist on calling the parents of the child who is hosting the party. It's really a good idea for you and your spouse to come to some agreement about the age at which a child would be permitted to go to parties where there are no adults present. Even more important, decisions have to be made about when it is okay to trust a child to go on a car date. Such conditions as meeting and becoming acquainted with the boy involved are essential. Again, we recognize that these are not simple matters; if the parents in the neighborhood could discuss these issues among themselves, life could be much easier. In lieu of this, your own family meetings can provide an important forum.

This, of course, raises the issue of when parents should allow their youngsters to begin dating, one of the all-time best-selling questions among parents and exceedingly difficult to answer. Age itself is not the critical factor. Some children at thirteen and fourteen are more mature than others at seventeen and eighteen. The kind of questions you should ask yourself would be: How old is the date? Have you met him or her? Can you meet the date's parents or at least call them? Will a car be used? Where are they going? What time will they come home? Are you reachable by phone if need be? And, especially, what is your own comfort level with regard to the specific dating situation?

Beyond all that, it's a good idea to have open discussions among your neighbors, the local PTA, and religious groups on what can reasonably be expected from children in your locality these days. We acknowledge being vague in our response to this subject, but frankly we prefer that both parents settle the issue on the basis of this kind of discussion rather than establish an arbitrary age rule that might not be appropriate for your situation.

• *It seems a lot of parents worry that their children will begin dating too young, but our problem is just the opposite. Our son is now seventeen and so far has shown almost no interest in girls. We've tried to encourage him to date, but he never responds and just shrugs it off. Does this mean there's something wrong with him?*
Here again the issue is not that he doesn't want to date—quite a few normal young men are simply not ready for dating—but rather, what else may or may not be happening in his life? How is his performance in school? Does he have friends? Does he pursue constructive leisure-time interests? Is it possible that his disinterest in dating is rooted in a feeling of inferiority and a fear that nobody will like him—a terror of rejection? If you suspect other complications, don't deal directly with the obvious issue of dating, but rather concern yourself with the possible underlying reasons for his problems, such as low self-esteem. You may decide that counseling or therapy is the best way to help your son resolve his underlying problems.

• *My wife and I simply can't get used to the idea that our fifteen-year-old daughter is calling boys up on the phone, sometimes even asking them if they want to see a movie with her. Is this kind of aggressive behavior common these days?*
To tell you the truth, the mother of the boy probably isn't happy about this situation, either. Those who grew up in the days when girls were not supposed to be so "forward" are sometimes chagrined by their daughters' behavior. It gets labeled "aggressive" because taking the initiative has traditionally been a male prerogative. Yet a girl calling a boy these days is usually not so much aggressive as *assertive* behavior. Among adults, such behavior is

becoming part of our culturally accepted norms, and adolescents tend to emulate what they observe in the older population. Things have changed; Sadie Hawkins Day used to be a once-a-year affair, but is now entering the mainstream of our daily lives.

Of course, it's possible for a girl to become openly aggressive in calling boys, making demands, even pushing for sexual relations with her boyfriend. This may disguise an underlying insecurity and a low self-esteem in girls who fear that if they don't make the move, no boy will be interested in them. In these situations parents might do well to explore their daughter's feelings in an understanding, helpful way. Criticizing your daughter or insisting that she stop will not be helpful (even if the behavior itself stops).

There is, however, nothing wrong with establishing rules about when and for how long your daughter can stay on the phone, especially if the family has only one number, or if getting homework completed is a problem.

• *My sixteen-year-old son has been dating a girl for about six months, and lately they have been seeing much less of each other. I suspect that sexual tension and pressures between them are at the heart of it, but I'm not sure how or if I should broach the subject with my son.*

This is a fairly common situation between adolescents. One of them (usually the boy) is pressuring the other to have sexual intercourse or to have more sexual contacts than the other feels comfortable with. Young people are often not well prepared to communicate about this problem between themselves, and the result is that the relationship goes downhill.

A concerned parent can make a neutral comment such as "I've noticed you haven't been seeing So-and-So lately—would you mind if I made some guesses as to the reason why?" and wait to see how the child responds. It's possible that the child won't want to discuss the issue, but chances are good that he or she can't talk to friends seriously about it and will welcome the opportunity for an adult viewpoint. Adolescents sometimes feel pressured to push for sex with a boyfriend or girlfriend when they're more interested in the broader aspects of the relationship and doing fun things together. Parents can explore the child's feelings about it and express their own feelings on the matter (without excessive moralizing).

• *I suspect that my fifteen-year-old daughter and her boyfriend are becoming sexually involved (although I don't think they've had intercourse). I've walked into the den a couple of times while they've been in there and it always seems as if they're buttoning up and straightening out their clothes. Should I say anything?*
While we believe strongly that adolescents of your daughter's age shouldn't have sexual intercourse, it's not such a simple matter when discussing other forms of sexual expression. This seems to be a matter for individual families to work out for themselves in terms of acceptable values and behaviors. Some parents feel that hugging and kissing, petting, and even mutual masturbation are acceptable forms of sexual discovery for adolescents. The problem is parents worry that, once their children start, they can't stop. Some parents, of course, don't want their children to engage in any sexually related activity. No matter what parents think about it, chances are their children will "make out."

We think you should talk to your daughter. However much we may have repeated this, we'd like to say again that talking about something is not license, permission, or encouragement. In fact, our best review of all the research on this subject reveals that young people who are able to talk with their parents about these intimate details are more likely to delay their first sexual experiences and, when they do have intercourse, to use contraception.

Parents have a much greater burden in sexuality education now that the vocal minority of zealots has deleted good programs or converted them to "abstinence-only" programs that deny reality, don't inform, and only preach. If we involve them, listen to them, and invite them to participate, we can help them ride the rapids of adolescence in one piece.

This is not to suggest that you go into intimate details. It's much wiser to have a general discussion, and to give what constitutes your best judgment.

• *For the third time in his high-school career, our son is going steady with a girlfriend (he's sixteen, she's fifteen and a half). It worries us somewhat how intensely attached he seems to get to these girls, and how crestfallen he is when they separate. Is this something most teenagers go through these days? The situation is now even more complicated, as they want to go on a weekend camping trip with some other steady couple. Should we put our foot down?*

Falling in and out of love is in fact a fairly common experience for young people. As we have suggested elsewhere, it's not a good idea to make fun of the youngster or in any way imply that it's part of his or her immaturity. Like everything else, going steady should be seen in context. Ask yourself if your son seems to be feeling good about himself and if there have been any deleterious changes in his normal behavior (eating, sleeping, doing chores, etc.) Once you put the question into perspective, you can decide how strict or trusting you want to be on related issues such as an overnight camping trip.

It seems perfectly legitimate to ask your son to hold off on that camping trip until a sense of trust and confidence has been established in the relationship between him and his steady girlfriend. You could say, "I'm not about to let you go on a trip as long as your schoolwork is in jeopardy," and so forth. The focus therefore is on the objective reality of the situation, rather than on whether or not you approve of his girlfriend or have some reservations about his going steady. The chances are that whatever you do will not be satisfactory to your son at this point. But that's where sticking to your best judgment counts.

• *My husband and I have just learned some very upsetting news. Our neighbor's son heard some boys talking about our sixteen-year-old daughter, and they were referring to her as a "slut" who'd put out for just about any boy who asked. We really love our daughter, and it really tears us up to think that she'd treat herself so badly. But we're afraid that if we say anything to her she'll feel we're accusing her. What if it isn't true?*

A lot of people think that the "sexual revolution" has eliminated the proverbial problem of a girl getting a "bad reputation," but this is not the case. Not only in small rural communities, but also in suburbs and cities, teenagers of both sexes circulate rumors (and occasional true stories) about who's willing to "do it." Parents need to be careful about how they handle any information, because sometimes "rumors" are started by insecure, boastful, or vengeful boys, or by jealous, insecure girls, and have little or no basis in reality. On the other hand, some girls do behave promiscuously. (We use the word "promiscuous" to refer to a series of self-damaging sexual experiences usually devoid of intimacy for the individual.) Very often the sexual behavior is compulsive and indicates very low self-esteem on the girl's part (boys too, of course, can be promiscuous, but they don't seem to suffer as much as the girls do from bad reputation).

In a situation such as yours there seems to us to be no substitute for confronting the problem and talking to your daughter without judgment. You could say, "Look, we were very worried. I'm sure if it were your own daughter, you would be, too." Or another possibility would be, "Let's see what we can do about the false rumor," even to the point of volunteering to call the parents of the boy or boys involved.

• *For the last two months my son has been seeing a girl whom neither my husband nor I like. She seems to come from a decent family, but her clothes are usually dirty, she uses a lot of profanity and is rude to us, and treats our son pretty badly as well (he*

doesn't object, however). We've tried to talk to him about this, but he simply refuses to consider our ideas and claims that we don't understand her or their relationship.
The situation of children bringing home "undesirables" is so common that it's one of the things parents fear most. With all their grand hopes for their children, parents are horrified when their daughter waltzes in with Rasputin, or their son becomes enamored of the Wicked Witch of the West. Parents have various objections—different religions, economic groups, political parties, sloppy, rude, childish, alcoholic, too old, too young, pregnant, unemployed, not college-bound, etc. Chances are that your evaluation is correct, from your point of view.

But your child doesn't see it that way and, besides, is in love.

Where do you go from here? What are your rights? You have a right to:

- Be enthusiastic or not
- Give your opinion or not
- Go along or fight it all the way
- Go to (and/or pay for) the wedding—or not
- Operate on the assumption that it won't last (your child will come to his or her senses)

You have these rights even though you don't *own* your children. Being a rigid authoritarian will either weaken or sever the connection between you. That's why it helps to avoid the following:

- Making the child more determined (young people have strong autonomy needs)
- Creating a confrontational atmosphere that propels your son or daughter into an antagonistic stance (sometimes the child gets carried away by the anger, and you then become the enemy)
- Focusing on your own reason for the opposition, whereas the overriding issue is whether it is a mature, loving relationship

We have heard of too many cases where young adults have, in retrospect, felt that their parents were right: "If only I had listened to them. But I couldn't. They were so mean, so insensitive, I was determined to have my own way."

Obviously, there are just as many circumstances where parents have been wrong and lived to regret it. Some were able to patch things up; some were not.

First, a few DON'Ts:

- Don't make it a test of wills.
- Don't start out by saying things like "How could you do this to me?" "After all I've done for you!" "When I was your age...."
- Don't break off relations.
- Don't say, "You'll get over it," "It's puppy love," "You can't be serious."

Now some DOs:

- Keep channels of communication open. (Listen and reflect with love and respect.)
- You must be civil to the person your child loves.
- Be polite. (It is a good way of maintaining distance and leaves the situation open for review.)
- Be welcoming. (If your child complains about your lack of enthusiasm, you say, "I have to be honest about my feelings, but our home is open to anyone who is your friend.")

Convey to your child that you know he or she will make up his/her own mind, and that you'll stand by him or her no matter what, but that you want to be heard.

Of course, if you are already in an antagonistic situation and have made some of the mistakes we've enumerated, it's going to be tough. But it may not be too late, especially if you acknowledge to your child that you were mistaken in your approach. It's a great first step toward trust and maturity in the relationship.

Ask your child to concentrate on whether the relationship is a mature one. (See the section on mature and immature relationships in Chapter 10, "For Teenagers and Young Adults.")

HOMOSEXUALITY

• *My wife and I have been in a panic ever since our son announced to us last week that he is a homosexual. How can a seventeen-year-old boy know himself well enough to even know what he is? We feel as if we've just lost our son.*

It is all right to hope that one's children will not grow up to be homosexuals. Because of discrimination and hostility, the life of a homosexual can be very difficult. And, of course, parents and other family members often suffer, believing that they have done something "wrong" that has contributed to the situation.

Our advice is to be perfectly sympathetic—no jokes, no derisive comments such as "You must be kidding" or "You'll get over it." Don't rush your child to a physician or a psychiatrist for "straightening out." The best first response is, "I'm so glad you feel free to tell us (me) about this. Let's talk. How long have you felt this way? How do you feel about it?" The point is to encourage a full and open discussion.

The child should be encouraged to be open-minded and to make no final decision about the matter until adulthood. Try not to give the message that homosexuality is evil or sinful: simply convey that the teenager is too young to decide. In any case, reassure the child that if he or she has had fantasies or even a pleasurable experience with a member of the same sex, this is not sufficient grounds for a lifetime decision. Experimental homosexual behavior, such as mutual masturbation, is common during the early adolescent years (ages eleven to fourteen or so), especially among boys. It is rarely a precursor of homosexuality in later life, and for most boys it is simply a developmental phase of their sexuality.

Some young people who declare themselves to be homosexual are rejected by their families. The rejection creates enormous problems; sometimes they become prostitutes (especially males).

Teenagers who "come out" typically encounter severe ostracism. Very few peer groups can tolerate this kind of acknowledgment. Yet some people would be greatly relieved if their sexual orientation were revealed. In some of the larger cities in this country gay and lesbian groups have provided clubs and recreational facilities for adolescents who want to identify themselves as homosexual. Some films, such as *Object of My Affection* and *Torch Song Trilogy,* have contributed to "lightening up" feelings about homosexuality. *Ellen* has brought the subject into our homes for discussion.

The following case study could be illuminating from a number of perspectives. An eighteen-year-old male student came to one of us and said, "I was one of your students. I need help. I have something terrible to confess. Can I trust you?"

He received the following response: "No."

He, in turn, responded, "What do you mean? You are supposed to be trusted."

"I know, but I don't know you. I don't know if I can be helpful. You don't know me. Trust comes only at the end of a relationship. All meaningful exchanges between people involve risk."

The student, getting the point, said, "Okay, I'll risk it. I'm a homosexual." The conversation continued as follows:

"Do you want to be a homosexual?"

"Of course not."

"Have you ever had a homosexual experience?"

"Of course not, what do you take me for?"

"I don't know yet. Have you ever had a heterosexual experience?"

"Of course not, I'm a homosexual. You're making fun of me."

"So far the diagnosis is asexual. Tell me your life history. You have five minutes."

As it turned out, he recalled having had homosexual fantasies at age twelve or thirteen. He didn't know that they were normal.

He felt overwhelmed with guilt, and he feared being "queer." The more guilt, the more compelling and more obsessive the thoughts; it became a self-fulfilling prophecy. Upon entering college, he searched for his identity in the index of a psychiatric textbook. It didn't help, because he had never had a homosexual experience, so he consulted an advanced psychiatric textbook, where he found the concept of latent homosexuality. He was then fully self-diagnosed, without having had any sex experience.

Our view is that there is no such thing as a latent homosexual. You might as well say that all women are latently pregnant. A person who is afraid of being homosexual or afraid of homosexuals isn't necessarily homosexual. It could just mean that the person is afraid.

This case history is important because there are many individuals who suffer from misinformation, teasing, harassment, and even murder. Peers often cruelly accuse people of being queer or gay for reasons related to popular stereotypes. The so-called effeminate male or "butch" female—blatant types who flaunt their homosexuality, often to protest the hostility of the "straight"—probably constitute only 5 percent of the homosexuals in our society. It is terribly important to support people who are harassed or in any way threatened by a peer group.

Society will have to accept the idea that it is okay to be a homosexual. If a person feels that he or she is gay, yet, at the same time, wants to fight it ("to be cured"), the initial rejection of homosexual feelings uses up most of the energy needed to effect the change. In a sense, one needs to say, "If I am, I am, but if I could figure a way out of it, I'd prefer it." The parents may want to say to the child—or preferably, think it—"I hope you aren't homosexual, but if you are, you remain my child. I will love you no less for it. I'm with you all the way." The part that must be verbalized is, **"I'm with you all the way."**

Despite all the research, no one really knows what the causes of homosexuality are. We deliberately state our position in this fashion because more and more research hasn't led to more and more understanding; in fact, it adds plausibility to the common-sense notion that the more we know, the less we know. We tend to be skeptical of researchers who "know."

Once upon a time, such researchers "knew" that if you had a weak father and a strong mother the chances of becoming a homosexual were pronounced. Most professionals in the field only recently discarded this theory. Apparently, researchers started out with the erroneous assumption that all homosexuals were in a state of arrested development. Lately, professionals have also taken another look at American families: it appears that *many* consist of strong mothers and weak fathers and most of them do not have homosexual children. In addition, virtually all the research on homosexuals has been done on patients in therapy. This would be analogous to concluding that heterosexuals are disturbed because more than 90 percent of people in therapy are heterosexual.

Only one thing is known with reasonable certainty: almost every homosexual was born to a heterosexual couple. The evidence of heredity, hormonal imbalance, and interactional patterns of parents is very sparse and lacking credibility.

Although cause remains a hotly debated issue, leading scholars have settled on the likelihood that a person's sexual orientation is pretty much determined by the age of four or five. Popular myths about the seduction and recruitment of children by homosexuals are disputed by the established research in the field. Arguments against hiring homosexual teachers are similarly questioned. In any case, more than 90 percent of all child molestation in schools involves heterosexual males and is directed at females. Should we bar heterosexual males from teaching in the public schools? Even if sexual identity were not determined by age five, it would be unrealistic to think that in a school where the teaching staff consists of 90 percent heterosexuals and 10 percent homosexuals, most of the children would flock to the latter. Are we eliminating heterosexuals as role models for children?

At one time professionals felt that people were *either* homosexual or heterosexual. Freud, however, postulated that all of us were born with a potential for bisexuality, capable of enjoying sexual experiences with either sex. Some writers in this field have even suggested that everyone would be bisexual if there were fewer social, moral, and legal prohibitions against it. We don't subscribe to the either/or theory and believe that the large majority of people are predominantly heterosexual, with perhaps 5 to 10 percent predominantly homosexual and 5 to 10 percent predominantly bisexual. Alfred Kinsey fairly well destroyed the either/or notion with his monumental research of the 1940s and 1950s. He suggested that people's sexual behavior could be categorized as follows:

0: Exclusively heterosexual behavior
1: Largely heterosexual but incidental homosexual behavior
2: Largely heterosexual but more than incidental homosexual behavior
3: Equal amounts of heterosexual and homosexual behavior
4: Largely homosexual but more than incidental heterosexual behavior
5: Largely homosexual behavior but incidental heterosexual behavior
6: Exclusively homosexual behavior

Kinsey's studies suggested that about 4 percent of males and 2 percent of females were probably exclusively homosexual. By the time they reach middle age, about 50 percent of males and 29 percent of females have had an overt erotic experience with a member of their own sex. He further suggested that 37 percent of all males and 13 percent of females had at least one homosexual experience to the point of orgasm between adolescence and old age. The Institute for Sexual Research founded by Alfred Kinsey has defined a homosexual as an adult who has had more than six sexual experiences with members of his or her own gender. On that basis, it is estimated that people with a predominantly homosexual orientation constitute about 10 percent of the population of the United States (more males than females). It has generally been estimated that about 30 percent of the homosexual population has "come out of the closet," that is, openly identified themselves as being gay.

Regarding rights and discrimination, we stand with the majority of well-informed people in the country who believe that people who happen to be homosexual are entitled to the same civil rights as heterosexuals. We strongly feel that any other position is simply bigotry.

We do not think that erotic desire and fantasy constitute the only elements in determining a person's sexuality. Our definition of a homosexual is, "A person who, in his or her *adult life,* has and prefers sexual relations with members of the same sex." A person could have many homosexual fantasies and experiences and still not be a homosexual. Masters and Johnson studies revealed that even exclusive heterosexuals acknowledge having homosexual fantasies. The idea that thoughts and even some experiences make one a homosexual could have a devastating impact on a person's life.

A true story might provide an appropriate illustration. Two fourteen-year-old boys regularly went to the attic after selling newspapers. There they would masturbate each other while looking at "girlie" magazines. On one occasion one of the boys picked up a male-body-builder magazine and looked at it. The other boy immediately said, "What's the matter with you, are you a faggot?" The fear that the partner might be homosexual negated the pleasurable experience. This story, described to us by one of our students, illustrates how ludicrous thinking can be about the topic. Both boys grew up heterosexual. Neither has been known to have any further homosexual interests or experiences.

Many parents do not have to deal with their child's homosexuality because most children simply do not confide in them.

Some parents prefer not to know. There are those who know and prefer to pretend they don't. We've heard of families whose children informed their parents of their homosexual orientation only to find out that the family couldn't cope with this knowledge. They interpreted this revelation as a rejection of everything they stood for, sometimes to the point of disinheriting their children, both financially and emotionally.

We also know families who developed a new family solidarity when a son or a daughter revealed a homosexual orientation. Parents should accept that being taken into confidence is a sign of trust, and should recognize, too, that it is psychologically better for the child to be able to acknowledge his or her sexual orientation rather than suffer a nagging worry about being "found out." For concerned parents, we recommend reading *Consenting Adult,* Laura Hobson's sensitive novel based on her personal experience. Also, get in touch with the National Gay and Lesbian Task Force [2320 17th St., N.W., Washington, D.C. The phone number is (202) 332-6483]. This group can put you in touch with other parents of gay children who are willing to serve in a supporting capacity. Another organization to benefit parents of gays is PARENTS FLAG (Parents and Friends of Lesbians and Gays), which has established parent groups throughout the country.

It is important to realize that most homosexuals manage well. They are mature, healthy people who are contributing, responsible members of society. Although significant numbers are neurotic, this can be said about heterosexuals as well. Perhaps one day a person's sexual orientation will be of no concern to anyone and people will be judged solely by their character and actions. We also should keep in mind that homosexuality is not a lifestyle—it is a sex style. Homosexuals exist in all walks of life. They espouse the same range of political and philosophical positions as are found among heterosexuals.

Homosexuals are more visible these days, yet no evidence exists to suggest that there are, in fact, more homosexuals. The real change lies in the fact that they are more open to discussion, and generally more accepting of themselves.[1]

• *Our thirteen-year-old son is very preoccupied with his male gym teacher. He is constantly talking about him, and it has reached the point where at least my husband is quite jealous. There are even times when my son tries to settle arguments based on his gym teacher's supposed opinion on the subject. We're not really concerned that our son is a homosexual, but we feel that his intense involvement may indicate some serious problems. He is also so involved in a sports training program that he shows no interest in having friends.*

We frequently encounter young adolescents having crushes on teachers of either sex, or engaging in hero worship (the idealization of movie stars or sports figures). Although these are not uncommon incidents and may represent a perfectly normal and passing phase, they could be problematic. Your son's situation doesn't seem too serious. The strategy should not be to attack the idol, but only the behavior about which you are concerned.

PORNOGRAPHY

• *My husband and I consider ourselves to be fairly open-minded but when it comes to our children, it's much harder to be objective. While cleaning my son's room this afternoon (he's fourteen), I found some pornographic magazines in his closet. I wasn't snooping, and the magazines weren't even well hidden. In a way it's funny, because I can remember reading anecdotes about mothers finding these things in their sons' rooms. But we're also worried—this wasn't just nudity, but hardcore pornography (some of the photos displayed people getting into bondage and discipline–sadomasochistic acts). Are these things harmful?*

---

1. In our judgment the best book for and about homosexuals is *Now That I'm Out, What Do I Do?* (paperback), by Brian McNaught.

Some people feel that if they are to succeed in instilling in their children a sense of sexual integrity, they must keep them away from pornography at all costs. Pornography is held up as the enemy of healthy adjustment, in the ranks of drug abuse and criminal behavior. We do not feel that pornography is appropriate for children (though we don't know how to stop them from seeing it). Most children at some point will encounter it or become interested for a time; even children with askable parents, from homes where sexuality has been openly discussed, may have their curiosity aroused by pornography.

Governments have often treated pornography as a social menace. This attitude has traditionally been based on the assumption that exposure to pornography has harmful effects on people. Furthermore, the legislatures of most Western countries have never been able to define it successfully. This task, for better or worse, has fallen to the courts.

Three basic theories exist to describe how pornography affects people. The first, or "modeling," theory argues that people imitate the sexual behavior that they witness in pornography. A second, or "cathartic" theory suggests that exposure to pornography *lessens* pent-up sexual drives, thus mitigating the possibility of antisocial or violent sexual behavior. The third, or "null," theory states that pornography has neither a stimulative nor a depressive effect on human sexual behavior.

Most contemporary research indicates that pornography is a symptom, not a cause of crime. [2] In this respect, the Danish experience is instructive. During the 1960s, Denmark experienced a rapid increase in the availability of pornography following its legalization. Sociological studies demonstrated that the overall

---

2. The 1985 Meese Commission on Pornography has been discredited by most of the legitimate researchers cited by it. Violence—not explicit sex—appears harmful. In any case, "causes" of rape and molestation are more likely to be found in experiences rooted in early childhood such as being molested by close relatives and parents. (See Oct. 1987 issue of *The American Psychologist.*)

number of sex crimes in Denmark *declined* in proportion to the *rising availability* of pornography. At this point it is premature to conclude that pornography lowered the number of sex crimes in Denmark. Other factors could be involved. Yet we can note that wide availability *did not* lead to an *increase* in any category of sexual offenses during the period under study.

Few psychiatrists believe that pornography causes individual pathology. Of the 3,423 psychiatrists who responded to a questionnaire on this subject, 80 percent reported never encountering an individual whose contact with pornography appeared to be a factor contributing to antisocial sexual behavior. Only 9 percent suspected such cases. About 7 percent were convinced they knew of such cases. Similar responses were received from professionals in child guidance, psychology, and social work. For instance, 77 percent of these individuals responded "No" to the question "Do you think reading obscene books plays a significant role in causing juvenile delinquency?"

We do not think that pornography is educational, but there are at least two persuasive arguments against banning adult access to it. The first has to do with "forbidden fruit." The second involves the constitutional right of adults to look at or read anything they want to. (We endorse laws that make it illegal to distribute pornography to juveniles.) It is of interest to note that December 1999 will mark the seventieth anniversary of the publication of Erskine Caldwell's *Tobacco Road*. Widely banned and considered pornographic at the time, it is now hailed as a significant contribution to American literature.

Our view is that if you ban pornography, you allow criminal elements that already control most of its production and distribution to earn more money. Anything that's banned immediately becomes more expensive and often more readily available. The more governmental regulation and restriction, the more possibility of organized criminal activity and control. Society should have learned a lesson from Prohibition.

["Pornography," in Webster's, is defined "as having little or no artistic merit" and is derived from a Greek word relating to "harlots." A syndicated *Baywatch* episode might well qualify; the main visual was a woman's derriere in a "thong" bathing suit while running down the beach, cheered on by giggles. Hardly a trace of artistic merit there (maybe it could provide a good discussion point for the difference between real life and TV)!]

The energy consumed in banning pornography would be better spent in establishing good sex education in our schools. We should deal with the problems that cause the desire for pornography, instead of focusing on the symptoms. Most antipornography activity is simply headline grabbing. People who are knowledgeable and relaxed about sex find pornography to be of little interest after a while. In fact, we think that a personal fixation on pornography is a symptom of emotional distress. We are not talking about readers of such magazines as *Playboy* or *Playgirl*. We mean pornography that degrades women and misuses children and especially pornography that *links sex to violence*. Pornography does not belong on billboards, the Internet, or television. Violence that is associated with sex is, in our view, more harmful to children than the grossest forms of pornography.

Here is an excerpt from a report by Sweden's State Commission on Aspects of Sex and Personal Relationships in Teaching and Public Education:

Teaching should systematically combat the picture of the relationship between man and woman promulgated by pornography and "sexism." The separation of sexuality and sexual life from the context of life at large and, particularly, the presentation of women purely as a sexual object, are incompatible with the objective proposed for sexual education.

Pornography is a symptom of society's unwillingness to promote responsible sexuality education at home and in the schools.

Now to return to the question of what (if anything) to say to your son. Without knowing your son it's hard to predict his reaction if you confront him with the "evidence," but it's a good guess that he might be embarrassed, guilty, angry, defensive, apologetic, frightened. On the other hand, he might have a healthy attitude about it, shrug it off, and inquire whether *you* have a hang-up. You and your husband might want to be alert to his possible sources for obtaining the materials; unless your son looks eighteen, few adult-bookstore proprietors would admit him. This would imply that some older person was obtaining the materials for your son or his peers.

When talking with your son, try an opening like this: "We realize that we're asking you to discuss a very private aspect of your life, but we've become concerned that you seem to be collecting pornography." This might help to alleviate some of the anxiety surrounding the conversation. Don't push him to discuss his feelings or accuse him of anything; you want to know because you care deeply about his well-being. (Incidentally, it might be wise for just one parent to broach this subject; two parents might be construed as an interrogation.)

Above all, be cautious lest you give your son the impression that he is "sick," and don't suggest that he should see a psychotherapist unless you suspect that he is fixated, i.e., that his involvement with pornography is becoming compulsive.

For the majority of adolescents who develop an interest in pornography, it is a passing involvement; hence, the suggestion that their curiosity is abnormal and "dirty" can do damage to their growing sense of identity. This is true also for addiction to soap operas and talk shows that focus on incest, abuse, and other destructively abnormal sexual areas. We prescribe patience for parents, especially if a child appears to be reasonably well adjusted in other areas.

LUST AND THE CONTEMPORARY
RELIGIOUS DILEMMA

• *My wife and I are conservative Christians, and we find it exceedingly difficult to tolerate what we feel are your permissive attitudes toward lust. We believe that they violate the religious principles we've tried to pass along to our children. We have a fifteen-year-old son, and we don't want him to act on all of his lustful feelings.*

Lust in men appears to be a near universal phenomenon, and in our society the prohibitions against it derive from Christ's pronouncement in Matthew 5:28: "But I say to you that every one who looks at a woman lustfully has already committed adultery with her in his heart." His message would seem to be clear, but contemporary theologians are now making a concerted effort to distinguish between *lust* and *fantasy*, two terms that have (erroneously) been used interchangeably.

A man who *lusts* after a woman (or another man) is pursuing a fantasy in an aggressive way; he meets her, his eyes scan her body, and he begins scheming ways to effect the seduction. His desire is his motivation. This is far from a developing relationship wherein sexual desire evolves in the context of the relationship itself. A man who *fantasizes* sexually about another person creates mental images in his mind and builds upon the scenario as he wishes. There is often little control over the appearance or disappearance of the thought itself, which may or may not be pleasurable to the individual. Day and night dreams that impinge upon us may involve being raped, ravaged, or witnessing one's own funeral, or they may be surreal and disconnected messages with no definite theme. The thoughts may be primitive symbols of the unconscious mind or may represent personal interest in a particular sexual situation. But they do not of themselves imply antisocial or sexist behavior, nor do they mean that the individual intends to live them out in real life. The theory that all dreams represent our real wishes is simply absurd. If a man accepts the fantasies as a healthy part of the personality, he will not suffer the obsessive repetition of the thoughts that are caused by guilt. For most men and women, the experience of both lust and fantasy can have physical as well as psychological ramifications. The stirring in the loins, the quickening pulse, and other physiological responses accompany the mental process. That doesn't matter. What matters is the behavior that results.

We can hardly imagine Christ's response to the images of lust that are thrust on our teenagers today! Global corporations have become increasingly bold in using lust to sell products, regardless of the harm to individuals and the planet. We are certain that teens express these images in some way, just as preschool children play-act the cartoons they see. Frank conversation and education allow teens to express in safe ways what they see and hear everywhere. It is especially hard for them to digest sexuality linked with violence, and as parents we must be alert to these and other references in their lives.

If anything, Christ was saying that lust is a distortion of man's instinctual sexual drive. It is a burden for women, who resent being "sex objects," and it can become a hypnotic force to the men preoccupied with it. In his book *Embodiment,* James B. Nelson states: "...if lust is untamed, inordinate sexual desire which is not only the passion for possession of another but which also becomes, by its centrality in the self, an expression of *idolatry,* then we are dealing here with something different from the usual erotic awareness expressed in sexual fantasy."

We would encourage you to view your son's behavior and attitudes using these guidelines, which, while maintaining respect and dignity for other human beings, do not seek to punish people for their sexual impulses alone. The book *Sex for Christians,* by Lewis B. Smedes, states: "Sensuous and sensual pleasure is good, and our desire for it is certainly not a distortion...Sensualism becomes a distortion of sexuality when it cuts physical pleasure in sex off from a personal quest for higher values. It distorts sexuality into a lust for physical pleasure that dominates one's sexual life."

For Teenagers
and Young Adults
(and Their Parents)

T *hese are questions* we have been asked many times by
young people over the past twenty-five years. You may find
that reading them will prepare you for questions your
younger brothers and sisters or other relatives might ask. At times
you may be helpful to your less-informed friends as well. Some
teenagers are more askable than their parents.

Would it surprise you to learn that the most frequently asked
question among young people is:

• *How can you tell if you're really in love?*
Why do so many people feel insecure about love? Why do people
fall in and out of it? Why do we hear so many complaints regarding regrets and mistakes about love? Why is it that, if you are a
teenager, adults (often parents) are quick to say, "It's puppy love,"
"You'll get over it," "Wait until you are older"? Can you fall in love
more than once? Is love at first sight worth much—or is it the best
kind? Is it true that love is blind? Our response is that if love is
blind, it had better not remain so for more than twenty-four hours.
After that, open your eyes and see the person in a clear light.

Raising a Child Responsibly in a Sexually Permissive World

If you feel yourself to be in love, *you are*. We're now referring only to the love for a special person, not for your parents, God, or a popular hero. We suspect that one can love many people but can be **in love** with only one person at a time.

Lots of people wonder how they can tell if they're really in love. Are there any signs? The answer is yes, but first you need to know that there are two essential kinds of love. We might think of them as **mature** and **immature** love. It's not that difficult to know whether love is mature or immature. Immature love is exhausting. You see people going around declaring, "I'm in love! I'm in love! I'm in love!" It's even exhausting watching them. They don't have time to shower, do their schoolwork, or help with household tasks. "How can I do the dishes? I'm in love!" Immature lovers often have what we call a hostile–dependent relationship. That means they don't enjoy being with those they supposedly love, yet they can't stand to be without them. When they're not with their partners, they miss them. But when they're together, they fight, argue, and act in a jealous manner.

What do you do when the person you love is always asking, "Do you love me? Do you love me?" Say no, explain why you said that, and you'll have your first genuine conversation.

When you are really in love, you enjoy it. Mature love is energizing. You have enough time and energy for most of the things you want to do. When you are with your loved one, you feel happy, joyous, and secure. That doesn't mean you never fight, but most of the time you really want to please the other person.

People still ask, "How can I tell if I'm really in love? What happens?" Some people actually think that they'll be hit by a thunderbolt. They wait their whole lives for this to happen. They go through many relationships looking for a "dream" person, that perfect someone who will live up to their fantasies. They don't realize that there is no such person.

Mature love is a slowly developing, exciting experience. Many relationships don't start out that way, but with effort and time

For Teenagers and Young Adults (and Their Parents)

they can become mature. The relationship does need to be mature before you settle down and take on shared responsibilities such as marriage and children.

Mature love is not motivated by a desire to be taken care of. If you feel you are nobody unless somebody takes care of you, you'll be nobody after somebody loves you. No one can validate who you are.

If you are really in love, you allow yourself to open up to the other person. Moving toward intimacy in this way involves a risk—that the other person may stop loving. You also accept mistakes, troubles, and periods of unhappiness. Many people think that sex is the most important part of love. This is not true. Caring deeply for another person is something quite apart from being turned on by a part of the body like a breast, a bicep, or a rear end.

If people can love each other in a mature way, they can make choices. They will marry for love.

How can you tell if you're really in love? By the energy you have.[1]

• What can I do if nobody likes me?

Maybe you believe that other people are responsible for your feelings, that others *make* you feel upset, hurt, angry, or happy. But, with the exception of physical pain, you make yourself feel just about every emotion you experience. Your way of thinking causes your emotions.

Self-acceptance has little to do with what other people think of you. With self-acceptance, you define yourself as worthy of existing. You just *are*. You are not the same as your behavior. Accept yourself and strive to change your behavior so that it expresses your best self.

Remember that each of us is a fallible human being. *All* human beings make mistakes. If you are able to apply this idea

1. For a fully elaborated explanation read *Why Love Is Not Enough* by Sol Gordon.

not only to yourself, but also to others, you will not need to engage in self-blame (guilt or anxiety) or other-blame (hostility).

People who are self-accepting are attractive to *some* other people. People who have poor self-esteem and express it in being (not looking) unattractive tend to repel rather than attract others.

If you feel depressed, the best way to get out of it is to do something that you really love to do and haven't done in a long time, or to learn something new. Or find a way to volunteer that gives you the feeling you're being of service to others. You *will* be more attractive when you have a vision of life as an opportunity rather than a burden! (If you want more ideas, read Sol Gordon's *Why Love Is Not Enough*).

• *Is it all right for teenagers to have sex?*

The odds are against it and the risks are too great. More than one million teenage girls get pregnant in the United States each year. Twelve million contract STDs (sexually transmitted disease—also called venereal disease, or VD). Each year many thousands of teenagers who have babies at age thirteen, fourteen, or fifteen lose the opportunities of adolescence and take on overwhelming responsibilities. In addition, they risk illness and possibly sterility (losing their capacity to have or father babies) because of untreated STD.

Unfortunately, in the past teenage girls fell rather easily for lines like "If you really love me, you'll have sex with me." Afterward, they were likely to be rejected and/or abandoned. We can hope that we are seeing a more enlightened time and adolescent females are becoming much more independent and strong.

Adolescence is a time for excitement, boy–girl get-togethers, and testing out relationships. Why spoil these opportunities to figure out what you want and need with a heavy sexual trip that almost no young person can handle? Sex is never a test of love. Only a period of mutual caring, of developing a trusting relationship, can reveal the true nature of love.

For Teenagers and Young Adults (and Their Parents)

It is difficult to imagine that any teenager—mature or otherwise—can handle the consequences of a pregnancy or the pain of developing a reputation for being "easy." We realize that teenagers are under a lot of pressure to conform, including from the media and the behavior of the adults around them, but don't kid yourself—most kids find that those early sexual experiences fail to live up to the "hype." Very seldom is it enjoyable, even though most young people won't admit it.

We feel it's better to wait until you are older. Older means at least eighteen, when you are away at college or working outside the home. At that age, young people have relatively easy access to birth-control methods and have had some experience with relationships. They can make some judgments about their readiness for sexual intercourse and take the time to have a fulfilling and mutually satisfying relationship first. They should know that it's even all right to wait until marriage.

Many young people find that they can be sexual with each other without having intercourse. A lot of young couples have discovered that they can be very sexual and loving with each other by hugging, kissing, and caressing.

We know what is often said: "Once you start, you can't stop." That's a lot of baloney. It's a line used mostly by boys for their own purposes. If a boy reaches his "peak of passion" and says he can't stop, all you have to say is, "I hear someone coming" (no pun intended). He'll stop on a dime.

We do know that some young people will have sex whether we like it or not and whether their parents like it or not. We advise them at least to use a reliable method of birth control, including condoms, which have the greatest chance of protecting against diseases that can be debilitating or fatal. It is wrong to bring an unwanted child into this world. It's not romantic to have sex without birth control, nor is it spontaneous. It's just plain stupid.

Of course, we know that there are some teenagers at sixteen or seventeen who have mature love affairs. Some are more mature than some adults. We still think they ought to wait. Maybe it seems unfair, but it is better to wait and "suffer a little" than to be sorry for a lifetime.

• *How can you tell if someone is handing you a line?*
If someone says, "If you really love me, you'll have sex with me," it's always a line. If that someone threatens to leave you if you don't (it's usually the boy telling the girl, but not always), then that person doesn't really care about you anyway.

Until such time as boys and girls stop playing games with each other, one should be prepared to play games in order to protect oneself. Here are some common lines with suggested answers:

HE: Let's go upstairs. I'd like to check your vault and perhaps make a deposit.

SHE: Your credit is no good. Take me home.

HE: Where have you been all my life?

SHE: Not waiting around for you.

HE: Where have you been hiding?

SHE: From you, dear.

HE: Would you like me to seduce you?

SHE: When I'm ready, I'll let you know.

HE: Would you like to get in the back seat of the car?

SHE: I prefer to sit up front with you.

HE: If we don't have sex, I'll go crazy.

SHE: Go.

HE: If you don't stay over, you'll never know what you're missing.

SHE: Yes, I know already.

HE: How can you do this to me?

SHE: You are doing it to yourself.

HE: You don't love me.

SHE: You are forcing me to have second thoughts about it.

HE: Don't worry, I'll use protection.

For *Teenagers and Young Adults (and Their Parents)*

SHE: You'll need protection if you don't leave me alone.
Here are some good ways of saying no:

- That's a line.
- No.
- I don't feel like it.
- No, it's against my religion.
- I have a headache.
- I don't know you well enough.

Finally, here is the ultimate line:

HE: I just oiled my machine. Want to see how it works?

SHE: (The ultimate put-down) Why don't you give it a cold shower and see if it rusts?

One day, people will realize that getting to know each other is truly the bottom line.

• *Do guys really respect you more if you say no?*

It would be easy for us to say, "Of course they do," and we'd be sure that you wouldn't believe us. The fact is that some do, and some don't. We feel very strongly that those who don't respect "no" care more about sex than they do about you. In many respects a good test of how much a male cares about you is his willingness to continue seeing you even if you don't have sex with him. What's really sad is when a girl feels that her only attraction is her sex appeal. Instead of promoting self-esteem, this leads to one exploitive situation after another. When boys are preoccupied with sex appeal instead of a relationship with a girl, they are invariably disappointed and look for somebody else who's closer to their fantasy. The dynamics here are usually that the boy feels inferior and is looking for a sex object to enhance his own self-esteem.

When you get right down to it, there's no substitute for a good friendship that might develop into a close love relationship.

• *How can you distinguish between possessiveness and love?*
Love is when you enjoy, respect, and appreciate another person.
Possessiveness is when you try to control and dominate another person. Excessive jealousy and anger are the chief signs of possessiveness.

• *I'm thinking about getting married. How can I be sure if it's the right thing to do?*
Don't if any of the following statements are true:

• When you are together, you spend most of your time disagreeing and quarreling.
• One of you is relentlessly asking, "Do you love me? Do you really love me?"
• You get bored spending a day together without watching TV.
• You feel he or she has traits you can't stand.
• He or she makes promises—like "Don't worry, when we get married I'll stop drinking (or stop fooling around)." If it's something you absolutely cannot tolerate, the person must make good on commitments *before* marriage. A bad situation usually gets worse after marriage.
• Your prospective mate insists that you drop all your old friends and start a whole new social life.
• You are getting married only to escape a bad home situation.
• You are under twenty years of age.
• You don't get along with one of your parents, and your prospective mate seems "just like" that troublesome parent.
• You've done some soul searching and discover you're marrying a "sex object."
• You disagree on whether or not to have children.
• You are being influenced mainly by the flattery or wealth of the in-laws-to-be.
• You don't agree on a basic lifestyle. Is it going to be a marriage of equals or a traditional marriage with the man as the "president" and the woman as "vice president"?

- You are of different religions and you can't agree on how the children should be raised.
- You don't plan to give your marriage priority over all else.

• Is it still considered normal to wait until marriage to have sex even though everyone else seems to have had sex already?

Yes, it's normal. No one should feel compelled to have sexual experiences before he or she is ready. It doesn't matter whether readiness is influenced by moral or religious reasons or simply by emotional maturity. A lot of people are intimidated by peer group pressure to have sex and often find themselves exploited by the experience and humiliated that they didn't stick to their own values.

On the other hand, no one should have unrealistic expectations about waiting until marriage. Waiting doesn't guarantee simultaneous, multiple orgasms. Most initial sexual experiences are not that exciting. In general, we need to understand that sexual compatibility is a learned process.

• Can you tell if a girl is a virgin?

A virgin is a person who has not had sexual intercourse.

The hymen, made of skin tissue, partially blocks the entrance to the vagina of many females who haven't had sexual intercourse. In quite a large number of females the hymen is ruptured as a result of exercise or masturbation, or for reasons that are not known. Often one cannot tell if a female is a virgin unless she is willing to tell you.

The first experience(s) of sexual intercourse can be painful for women. Sometimes, but not always, there can be some bleeding. Gentleness in initial insertion is important.

Some boys who boast about having many partners say that when they marry they will marry virgins. Our response is we hope you'll marry a person, not a hymen. Only men who are themselves virgins are entitled to expect the same of their brides.

Raising a Child Responsibly in a Sexually Permissive World

• *My girlfriend and I have been dating for four years. She is the only sexual partner I have had. Do you think I should have sex with someone else before I get married to her?*
What would be the point of having sex with someone else? The opportunities for variety are endless, even with one person. Why risk spoiling the relationship?

• *Is it all right for females to be assertive?*
Assertiveness is a good quality. It means that you know what your goals are and you strive to obtain them. It means learning how to stand up for your rights even in uncomfortable situations. (Assertiveness is different from being aggressive. Aggressiveness is being insensitive to the rights of others.)

A good exercise suggested by our colleague, Oralee Wachter, is to develop Your Bill of Rights.

Here are some suggestions:

I have a right to

change my mind;
say I don't feel like it;
be responsible for my own sexual feelings;
ask for what I want;
enjoy hugging and kissing without it meaning that I want sex;
not act macho;
refuse a date without feeling guilty;
say no;
say yes.

You also have a right to be free of constant bombardment by sexual innuendo and titillation from the media. You have the right to up-to-date knowledge on sexuality and contraception and disease-prevention. You have the right to be educated on the responsibilities of parenting.

What are some rights you would like to add?
I have a right to

1.

2.

3.

4.

5.

6.

7.

8.

• *Do men enjoy and/or appreciate initiation of sexual friendships by women?*
Many men do these days.

NORMAL/ABNORMAL

• *Is there a way of telling what is normal or abnormal sex between two people?*
Generally speaking, normal behavior is voluntary (both people consent to it). This behavior is not exploitive. It is free of guilt and serves to enrich the relationship. Abnormal behavior tends to be driven or compulsive. It has a tendency to hurt another person. It is usually selfish and exploitive.

• *Why do people have sex hang-ups in the first place?*
Hang-ups are cultural, passed from parents to children, and picked up from society. If you aren't hung up about sex, chances are your children won't be.

• *What about your thoughts?*
What you *do* counts, not what you think. All thoughts are normal, no matter how weird. Difficulty arises if you feel guilty about a thought. Then you'll keep having it. Guilt is the energy for the repetition of unacceptable thoughts.

• *Are sexual fantasies normal during intercourse?*
Sexual fantasies are normal and common, and for some people they provide an added zest to the experience.

• *Why is it easier for males to have intercourse without emotional involvement than it is for most females?*
Contrary to popular belief, it is just as enjoyable for men to be emotionally involved as for women. Unfortunately, there are still too many men who are responsive to the double standard and the expectations of the sexist society in which we live. They don't seem to be happier for it. With the growing impact of the feminist movement, this kind of question will ideally become obsolete.

• *Why is it that men and women always seem to get involved in power struggles over sex? It seems that men are always trying to have sex more than their partners want it.*
The joke you'll hear most often about this situation goes something like "Not tonight, dear—I have a headache." It's been suggested that such apparent differences in sex drives are due mainly to biological (hormonal) forces, and that they thus represent "natural" variations between the sexes. We don't agree with this point of view.

We believe that sexual desire is primarily a psychological phenomenon, affected by many forces. In our society, men are programmed to feel they need sex; to men, intimacy, closeness, and touching are equated with sexual intercourse. Thus, when a woman expresses a desire for closeness, the male often assumes that this means she wants intercourse (when what she really might want is to cuddle). At times it does appear as if a power struggle exists, in large part because there is often little or no communication between the partners about their desires.

Women's programming also plays a role in the conflict. Women tend to be raised to believe that sex is dangerous, and the "men are after only one thing." Thus, they might tend to resist sex without knowing why (just as men might pursue sex without really feeling like it—what they really want might be cuddling or massage). Who knows how much cultural indoctrination plays a part here, with sex depicted so casually rather than integrated into loving relationships.

• *I'm an eighteen-year-old girl and I've never reached an orgasm. Am I normal?*
Whether you have orgasms or not has little or nothing to do with being normal. What you need to know is that very few teenage women achieve orgasm the first times they have sex. Many will even acknowledge that sex isn't that great in its initial stages. Good sex has to do with shared intimacies, practice, and feeling loved. Many women reach their first orgasm through masturbation, and some through mutual masturbation.

• *Is it true that "normal" people need sex every two or three days? Is it normal in a loving relationship to be satisfied with sex once a week?*
There is no such thing as a normal rate of sexual intercourse. Some enjoy it frequently and others infrequently. What counts is what's mutually satisfying. Of course you can have a satisfactory relationship having sex once a week.

Raising a Child Responsibly in a Sexually Permissive World

• *Does the size of one's penis make a difference?*
No. Besides, you can't tell the size of an erect penis from observing its flaccid state. A lot of males worry because their penis seems small when compared with others'. What they don't know is that in an erect state their penis could be larger than those that appear huge in a nonerect state. A girl doesn't need to be concerned that a particular penis is too large for her. The vagina adjusts to any size penis.

• *Can you still be normal sexually if you have an aversion to oral or anal sex?*
People should be free to have any kind of sexual preference. There may be some problems if a person finds this experience revolting or disgusting. On the other hand, many people have perfectly normal, healthy sexual experiences without either oral or anal sex. They are, however, increasingly becoming part of the repertoire of sexually compatible couples. (There is now an AIDS risk. See Chapter 11).

• *What would you think about a person who doesn't seem to need sex at all? I'm a male senior, I've never had sex, I don't masturbate. I'm happy, I'm successful, but sex of any kind does not interest me personally. Do you think I'm normal?*
There is not necessarily anything wrong with someone who feels the way you do. Just as in the same way there's nothing wrong with anybody who decides to be celibate for the rest of his or her life, as is required in some religious orders. You can always change your mind and enter into sexual relationships at a later time in your life. If you are not happy about your low sex drive, or you suspect that there is some physical cause, you may want to seek professional guidance.

• *What about masturbation?*
It is normal and healthy for both males and females. No physical harm results even if you think you are doing it too much. Males don't have to worry that they will run out of sperm; a fresh supply

is readily available. You need be concerned only if you seem to masturbate compulsively—that is, if you "can't help yourself" and don't enjoy the experience. Guilt is usually the energy behind compulsive masturbation.

SEXUAL RELATIONSHIPS

• *Do males and females have cycles during which they feel more sexual than at other times?*
We think sex has larger psychological components than physiological ones. Your relative state of sexual desire depends more on your mood and state of mind than on physical or hormonal cycles.

• *How can I start a sexual dialogue with a man so that he will respond to my individual needs?*
Try something like this: "Can I tell you some things about my sexual feelings, which you could not possibly know about, unless I told you?" His response will be, "Sure." Then lay it on him (but without being critical).

• *How can a girl tell if she has an orgasm?*
Orgasm is most often associated with pleasurable sensations related to the clitoris. But women can achieve orgasm from a wide range of sexual stimulations. A good way to think about orgasm is as a peak experience, intensely pleasurable, and then a nice relaxed feeling afterward. Women who have not experienced orgasms are often encouraged to masturbate as a good way to learn.

• *Is it possible for a woman to achieve orgasm without the clitoris being stimulated?*
Yes.

• *I find direct clitoral stimulation painful.*
Some women do. Many women prefer indirect stimulation.

• *Is there a difference between ejaculation and orgasm in the male?*
Yes, ejaculation can occur without orgasm. Orgasm, however, is usually accompanied by ejaculation in males. This is not generally acknowledged, but men realize there is a big difference in the intensity of orgasm at different times.

• *What is the best way to prevent ejaculation from happening immediately after entering the vagina?*
It is not unusual, during the first few times a man has sex or when circumstances are anxiety-filled, to have a premature ejaculation. If the problem is not solved soon enough for you, it could be due to fear of failure. A couple should then experiment with being together sexually for a few weeks without having sexual intercourse. Get to feel comfortable with each other without the need to "perform." Another approach that works with some males is to masturbate an hour or so before having sexual intercourse; some males last longer the second time around.

In any case, if the premature ejaculation persists, a sex counselor should be consulted, or, if you prefer, first read one of the books recommended in the bibliography to see if the advice works for you.

• *When I have sex and come, it takes me a long time, perhaps half an hour, before I can get hard again. Does that mean there is something wrong with me?*
No. It's called the refractory period. It takes a while for males to achieve an erection after ejaculating.

• *How can you persuade your partner to participate in oral sex?*
You can try to encourage your partner by suggesting that if he or she does not enjoy it you would not apply any more pressure. There are perfectly normal people who don't enjoy oral sex. (In any case, we advise against oral sex unless you are monogamous partners.)

For Teenagers and Young Adults (and Their Parents)

• *Do pot, alcohol, or other drugs act as a sexual stimulant?*
Communicating with another person is a much better way to
heighten sexuality. Drugs may result in an artificial stimulation of
certain senses, but they also tend to turn you in on yourself, thus
cutting off the other person. Drugs dilute the experience. With
alcohol, more than just a small amount tends to inhibit sexual
responsiveness.

HOMOSEXUALITY

• *How can you tell if a person is homosexual?*
You can't unless they say so. People simply are what they are. No
one chooses to be a homosexual. Therefore, it is not okay to be
antigay. This is true in the same respect that it is not okay to be
anti–people who are left-handed.

A lot of young people worry about their own impulses. Many
have homosexual thoughts or even a few experiences. This does
not make them homosexual. A homosexual is a person who as an
adult prefers relations with members of the same sex.

A young person might be approached by an adult homosexual—but much more often by an adult heterosexual—for the
wrong reasons. The response should be, "No, thank you." Just
walk away. The vast majority of homosexuals are just like the
majority of heterosexuals. They do not try to seduce young people. Furthermore, they are pretty discreet about their own sexual
behavior. That's why you can't tell whether or not a person is
homosexual just by observing behavior. Only a small number are
deliberately effeminate (or masculine in the case of lesbians) and
put on a "show," mainly to annoy people in a society that dis-
criminates against homosexuals.

• *What causes a person to be homosexual?*
The causes of homosexuality remain unknown. Evidence suggests that a person's sexual orientation is determined by the time
they are five years old. Sexuality, whether it is heterosexual or

homosexual, can be considered abnormal only if it is exploitive or self-destructive.

• *A friend of mine recently announced that he is a homosexual, and I'm having trouble deciding if I can remain friends with him.*

This is a fairly common situation and one that sometimes threatens people. Sometimes, the person to whom the news is revealed fears that the gay person will make a sexual overture. Although this is sometimes the case, usually the gay person divulged this personal information because he or she had grown uncomfortable with the secrecy and pretense of hiding their true identity.

Despite substantial improvements in the last decade, popular polls and recent municipal elections suggest that a significant minority of Americans do not approve of gay rights. Our Constitution was designed to protect the basic rights of a minority, even if a majority does not approve. If our black population had to wait for a majority of people in the country to accept "equality of all before the law," we would still be where we were before the landmark Civil Rights Act of the sixties. Instead there were courageous demonstrations, creative and powerful "events" such as boycotts, and other political struggles and shows such as *Roots* and *All in the Family*.

It is all right to have your personal opinion about homosexuality. Violence against people based on their sexual preferences is totally unacceptable. It should be a national priority to eradicate such harassment and murder. What consenting adults do in private is no one's business. There is something wrong with people who intrude into other people's private affairs. The people for whom we have the least respect are those who use the Bible to justify their hatred or bigotry. God's message to all of us is to "love thy neighbor as thyself."

• *As a female, I am constantly intrigued (turned on) by the female body, including my own. However, I don't relate this to my sexual preference. In fact, it increases my sexual desire for a man (I think). Is this possible? Or does this type of arousal indicate homosexual orientation?*

This is such a common feeling, but very few boys or girls are willing to acknowledge it to anyone else. Why shouldn't a body be a turn-on? It does not reveal a homosexual orientation. We're not suggesting that turn-ons represent an invitation to exploitation or are substitutes for relationships. It could just be a nice feeling. Homosexuality refers to a desire to have sexual relations only with members of the same sex.

CONTRACEPTION, PREGNANCY, STDS

• *Is the pill harmful?*

As of this writing, the pill is still reported safe if taken under the direction of a doctor. Women with histories of diabetes, heart disease, liver malfunction, migraine headaches, high blood pressure, cancer, or those over 40 who smoke should not be on the pill. Check with your doctor. Some recent studies of the pill have suggested links to breast cancer, but this link has not been definitively determined. As a consequence, more and more women are using the diaphragm. Until more research is provided, teenagers would be safer using this or other forms of contraception.

• *What's the best method of birth control for people who are just starting out to have sex?*

The best protection is for the male to use a *latex condom with nonoxynol-9* and the female a contraceptive foam with a spermicide. Neither requires a prescription. Both are available from most drugstores. Follow the directions on the labels. Both are necessary for protection against STD, as well as against unwanted pregnancy.

• *Are there any new methods of birth control coming out for men?*
Yes, but a male pill is still in the future. The condom and a vasectomy (sterilization) are still the only two choices.

• *What effect does having a vasectomy have on your sex life?*
Vasectomy is a procedure to prevent the release of sperm when the male ejaculates. It is a simple operation that is done on an outpatient basis and has no ill effect on the sex life. As a matter of fact, many males report that their sex lives improve because there is no fear of impregnating their partner.

• *Is there any "safe" way or time to have sex without practicing birth control?*
Don't believe stories that you can't get pregnant if you have sex standing up, or if it's the first time, or if you've taken one pill, or if he pulled out in time. Withdrawal is not a good method because a few drops of semen are released from the penis before ejaculation, and these few drops contain sperm that can impregnate. Anytime you have unprotected sexual intercourse you risk pregnancy. Even though the risk is less a day or two before, during, and after the period, there is still a risk.

• *Is it safe for a pregnant woman to have intercourse?*
Generally speaking, it is safe for pregnant women to have intercourse. Some women find that they don't feel like having sex during this time, while others find that pregnancy heightens their sexual desires. Men should be sensitive to these feelings.

Some new evidence, however, suggests that some women should avoid intercourse during the last trimester (three months) of pregnancy. This is especially the case for women with a history of miscarriages or with premature ripening of the cervix, something your doctor can diagnose. Recent, but not definitive, medical studies also suggest that *all* women should avoid intercourse in the last month of pregnancy because of a slight chance of triggering an

For Teenagers and Young Adults (and Their Parents)

early labor. An obstetrician would be able to advise each woman what is best for her.

• *Is it possible to become pregnant without intercourse—that is, from sperm ejaculated right outside the vagina?*
Yes, but it is rare. It is also very rare for a girl to get pregnant from sperm on a guy's fingers.

• *How does rhythm work? What are the safest days for having intercourse?*
The safest days for having intercourse are a couple of days before a female's menstrual period, during the period itself, and a couple of days after. Ovulation occurs about fourteen days before the onset of the next period; because of irregularities in women's cycles, this is impossible to predict with absolute certainty. It is now believed that every time a woman has unprotected intercourse she risks pregnancy. One way to become a parent is to rely on the rhythm method.

However, much scientific work is being done in this area of "natural" family planning; perhaps a reliable natural method of birth control will someday be available.

• *How many weeks after conception is it still relatively safe to have an abortion?*
The earlier you have an abortion, the safer it is. To be legal, in most cases, it must be done before the twenty-fourth week. If it is performed within the first twelve weeks, there is less physical risk than childbirth and it is less traumatic. For most women the psychological repercussions of abortion are also less than those of an unwanted birth.

• *Is it safe for a woman to have more than one abortion?*
Generally speaking it is safe—much safer than childbirth—for a woman to have one or two abortions. However, multiple abortions

(more than four) can jeopardize a woman's future chances of carrying a baby to term. Abortion should never be used as a form of birth control.

• *Is herpes as bad as everybody is saying it is?*

The severity of physical symptoms varies from person to person. In some people, the blisters and pain are acute and last for a relatively long time, while in other people the symptoms are mild and go away quickly. Some people have frequent recurrences, while others never experience an outbreak again.

We assume you're asking about the psychological effects of contracting a sexually transmitted disease that cannot, as of now, be cured. The media have even referred to herpes sufferers as the "new lepers." We feel that while the *initial* shock of contracting herpes can be severe, most people recover and adjust well to the situation. Many of them marry and have children (though here medical precautions must be observed).

Within any relationships, the main factor is honesty: if you have herpes, tell any prospective partner the truth *before* having sexual relations. People who have herpes find that few partners reject them sexually for that reason alone.

• *Can you get STD more than once?*

Yes, you can be reinfected any time you are cured of previous infections. You can also have more than one STD at a time.

• *How can you tell if you have gonorrhea?*

Gonorrhea usually shows up in men two to six days after sexual contact with an infected person. In some cases, it doesn't show up for a month or more. The first sign is usually pus dripping from the penis or a burning feeling while urinating. However, about 10 percent of the men who get gonorrhea show no signs at all. Just the same, the disease can be spreading through their bodies, and anyone who has sex with them is likely to become infected.

If gonorrhea remains untreated, it can cause sterility, arthritis, heart trouble, and general bad health. Treatment at any public health clinic is confidential and not subject to parental approval.

FERTILITY

• *Are many couples infertile, and is science making progress in this area?*

It is estimated that there are in the United States about ten million adults between the ages of eighteen and forty who experience difficulties in conceiving a child or carrying a pregnancy to term. Infertility is on the rise because of sexually transmitted disease, a tendency to postpone childbearing, and many other unknown factors. Medical science continues to make slow but steady progress to assist couples who are finding it difficult to conceive. (The rise of multiple births in conjunction with the use of aggressive fertility technologies is now posing bioethical questions). When a woman is unable to conceive, we call her infertile. There can be several reasons. Her fallopian tubes may be blocked so the egg (ovum) necessary for fertilization does not descend. There may be a hormonal imbalance or other medical reasons. If a woman wishes to have a child but does not get pregnant, she should consult a physician who specializes in that field. Sometimes there are psychological reasons for inability to conceive. Psychotherapy can then be of help. Childlessness, of course, cannot always be attributed to the woman. A significant number of men are sterile—i.e., their sperm is unable to fertilize the egg. A physician can diagnose sterility through a sperm count and analysis. If a couple have been unable to conceive, the male should be examined first, because his examination is relatively simple and inexpensive.

C H A P T E R   E L E V E N

STD—*Sexually Transmitted Diseases*

O*ne of the most pressing areas* in the entire field of human sexuality and, at the same time, one of the topics enveloped by ignorance and misinformation is venereal disease, now referred to as sexually transmitted disease (STD). Read the following four statements and decide whether each is true or false.

1. Syphilis and gonorrhea are the only serious venereal diseases in the United States.
2. STD can be transmitted only via genital contact.
3. Once the signs of STD disappear, the person is cured.
4. Once you contract STD, you certainly know you have it.

All four statements are false. Most young people—and even most adults—would answer "True" to one or more of these statements, a dramatic illustration of how much education is needed to help people recognize the dangers of STD. Every parent should be well informed on this topic—it's a matter of life and death. In a survey done by the Kaiser Family foundation, only 23% of respondents listed chlamydia as an STD, and yet it's the most common STD in the United States.

The United States Public Health Service's Center for Disease Control estimates that at least 12 million Americans contract a form of sexually transmitted disease each year (the highest in the world). The annual medical cost of this disease is staggering: about $1 billion. The emotional trauma suffered by afflicted individuals, as well as the strains it places on relationships, can hardly be measured. Sexually transmitted disease now constitutes the number-one reportable communicable disease in the United States. The problem is most serious among young adults, where the STD rate in the sixteen-to-twenty age group is three times the level in the general population.

The breadth and seriousness of venereal disease in the United States have led many researchers and educators to redefine the entire area of study. In fact, the term "venereal disease" refers most directly to diseases contracted during sexual intercourse. Because many infections can be transmitted during other intimate body contacts, the preferred term is STD—i.e., diseases that are capable of being transmitted through contact with the genitals, the anus, the mouth, and other body areas.

Some believe that this epidemic results from increased sexual promiscuity, ignorance, or professional and public apathy. Whether you agree or not, the fact remains that the available statistics are shocking.

Here are the estimated annual incidences of new cases of sexually transmitted diseases: chlamydia, 4 million; gonorrhea, 800,000; condyloma (genital warts), 1 million; genital herpes, 500,000; syphilis, 101,000; HIV, 80,000; PID, 1 million; trichomoniasis, 3 million; and hepatitis B, 200,000. As reported in the *New York Times*, Nov. 24, 1998, 3 million adolescents a year contract an STD—a clear indication of unsafe sex that also increases the risk of transmitting HIV.

Chlamydia and condyloma have replaced genital herpes as the new raging epidemics. Condyloma is a virus that breeds in the warm, moist tissues of the genital tract and causes cauliflowerlike warts. Antibiotics do not kill the growths, and the warts must be removed. Condyloma's favorite targets are fifteen to twenty five year olds.

The most serious and tragic of all STDs is AIDS—a fatal disease which had caused as many as 400,000 deaths in the United States by the end of 1998.[1] Since 1981, when AIDS was first recognized, 47 million people have become infected and 14 million have died worldwide. All but 5 percent of the infections occurred in Asia, Africa, and Eastern Europe. (Source—UNAIDS, 1998.)

It is important to understand that STD refers to a wide range of diseases, including but not limited to syphilis, gonorrhea, NGU, genital herpes, and AIDS. In fact, there are twelve diseases in addition to the commonly recognized venereal ones (syphilis and gonorrhea) that qualify as STDs. In this section we'll discuss briefly each of the important ones. We provide this information out of our strong conviction that knowledge promotes responsible behavior; conversely, ignorance of the methods of STD prevention and detection can potentially harm the individual's health and well-being. When someone suspects that he or she is infected with an STD, competent medical diagnosis and treatment must be sought. **Home remedies should not be attempted** and may serve only to complicate matters.

SYPHILIS

Syphilis is almost always spread by some form of sexual contact. We say "almost always" because some people might not think of kissing as sexual. There have been occasional cases where a person has caught the disease by open-mouth kissing with someone who had it.

Left untreated, syphilis can last for a person's lifetime. There are thousands of infected people who aren't aware of having it; either

---

1. The AIDS virus does not directly kill anyone but destroys the immune system—leaving infected people vulnerable to other fatal conditions. More than a million Americans, including women and children, are believed to be infected by the AIDS virus. Most are symptom-free, but the Surgeon General's office estimates that as many as one-third will develop an illness that will prove fatal within five to ten years.

they were never treated, or they think they no longer have the disease. Untreated, syphilis can result in serious disabilities, including paralysis, brain injury and insanity, heart disease, and skin disease.

Syphilis can be detected and successfully treated by a physician. The drug of choice is penicillin, unless the individual is allergic to it, in which case synthetic antibiotics are prescribed. Any damage already done by the disease cannot be reversed. Thus, the importance of early diagnosis and treatment is obvious, for even though the spirochete bacteria that cause syphilis may have been killed, a damaged heart will never regenerate.

It is important to remember that syphilis goes through three main stages. The first stage is usually signaled by the appearance of a sore called a chancre. It appears anywhere from ten to ninety days after the bacteria enter the body. The sore resembles a pimple or wart and may or may not produce pus. In men it usually appears on the penis. In women it usually shows up either on the labia or inside the vagina. The chancre produces neither pain nor itching and, especially among women, may go undetected if not visible. Chancres may appear in other places on the body where sexual contact was made, in an odd spot (on the arm or a toe), or simply not at all.

The second stage of the disease begins with the disappearance of sores. This does not signal a cure. From about two weeks to six months after the initial contact, other signs (a rash; welts around the genitals; ugly sores in the armpits, between the toes, or in the mouth; a low-grade fever; headaches; sore throat) make themselves known. These symptoms are sometimes attributable to other, less serious causes and may disappear and recur in some people. Eventually, in all victims they disappear.

A patient usually enters the third stage of syphilis about two years after initially contracting the disease. While still infected, the person is no longer infectious; the illness cannot be passed to another person. The one exception to this rule is a pregnant woman, who can pass the infection on to her fetus. An individual can feel quite healthy during this stage of the illness, but the infection continues to do more and more damage. During the next five years, the disease will probably affect the heart, the brain, and other organs, ultimately causing both physical and mental crippling and possibly death. About 400,000 people a year contract syphilis in the United States.

GONORRHEA

Gonorrhea has been popularly known by many names: "the clap," "the drip," "a dose," "the whites," "morning drop," and other colloquialisms. Myths that some people have believed are that you can contract gonorrhea from lifting something heavy or from contact with toilet seats, doorknobs, dirty sheets, and unwashed eating utensils.

A person contracts gonorrhea in almost all cases when the penis enters the vagina, the mouth, or the rectum. Gonorrhea bacteria (gonococci) thrive in the type of tissue found in the urinary tract, the throat, the cervix, and the rectum. The disease has a number of potentially dangerous results. Untreated gonorrhea is the most common cause of sterility in women. It can cause arthritis, heart disease, and general poor health. Men who have had gonorrhea sometimes have difficulty urinating for the remainder of their lives. As is the case with syphilis, gonorrhea can be detected and successfully treated. An individual can contract the disease as many times as he or she comes into contact with another infected person.

Between three and six days after the gonococci enter the body, a man usually experiences a milky-white drip from the penis, which may be accompanied by a burning sensation when urinating. Occasionally these signs don't appear until about a month after the initial contact. Furthermore, in some cases a large amount of pus may be discharged. In other cases, a male will notice only a slight, cloudy discharge in the morning. The burning feeling while urinating may be only a little uncomfortable, or it may be extremely painful. It is important to note that about 10 to 20 percent of males who contract gonorrhea show minor symptoms or no signs at all. Among women, there may be a slight discharge from the vagina along with a burning feeling, but 80 percent of the time there are no symptoms. Thus, a woman may not know she has contracted gonorrhea for weeks, months, or even years after she has initially been infected.

As of this date the medical tests for the detection of gonorrhea are not completely reliable, particularly for women in the first stages of the illness. As the disease progresses, the tests become more accurate. For this reason, sexually active people who have more than one partner should be regularly tested for gonorrhea whether or not they think they have it. This is particularly important in light of the fact that, as with syphilis, the symptoms of gonorrhea can disappear even without medical treatment. All the while, the disease is damaging the body. About 3 million people in the United States are infected with gonorrhea each year.

NGU (NONGONOCOCCAL URETHRITIS)

According to the Center for Disease Control, NGU has quickly become a major national health problem. Actually, it has been with us for a long time. Its symptoms can be misleading; they also tend to show signs of fading away and may not be easily recognized by some physicians. Unlike other STDs such as gonorrhea and syphilis, NGU is still not considered a communicable disease that must be reported.

The bacterium *Chlamydis trachomatis* causes about one-half of all NGU cases. The remainder is attributable to other organisms and irritation. NGU occurs most frequently in the urethra, the tube that runs from the bladder through the penis, or to the urethral opening in women. The disease generates pus in this area and thus in some respects resembles gonorrhea. NGU can cause an infection in the male's sperm ducts, sometimes causing a "drip," and can cause sterility if left unchecked. Another result may be prostatitis, a disorder of the prostate gland. Unchecked NGU in women may possibly cause sterility. Furthermore, NGU can attack newborn babies and cause pneumonia and eye infections; numerous stillborn deaths are blamed on NGU. Luckily, as with gonorrhea and syphilis, NGU can be successfully treated with antibiotics.

GENITAL HERPES

There are two types of herpes viruses. Type 1 appears most frequently on the lips. Type 2, or herpes simplex, occurs most frequently in the genital area, though each can occur in either location and can be transferred from one part of the body to another by touching. Type 2, genital herpes, is almost always a sexually transmitted disease.

No cure for genital herpes exists at this time. A new medication being introduced, however, promises relief of the symptoms of the first outbreak of the virus. The medication is called acyclovir, also known as ACV and Zovirax. It is available in capsules, tablets, suspension (for oral use), ointment, and powder (for IV use). Researchers emphasize that the new medication is not a cure and is effective mainly against the symptoms of the initial outbreak. Thus, the real hope lies in prevention—and communication serves as our best line of defense.

The visible signs of genital herpes will appear very shortly after the initial contact, perhaps as quickly as one or two days. For women, the first experience of the disease will last about three weeks; the sores usually are very painful and are accompanied by flulike symptoms such as fever and headaches; then the disease enters a latent stage. For men, the first episode is somewhat shorter, perhaps two weeks, and the symptoms are somewhat less severe. In both men and women genital herpes usually reappears, although in later episodes the symptoms may be less severe than in the first one. These recurrences may be quite irregular and, perhaps, happen during periods of stress.

The seriousness of herpes is appreciated only when looking at the broader picture. At present, a person who contracts herpes is infected for an entire lifetime. Researchers have discovered that herpes increases a woman's chances of developing cervical cancer.

Furthermore, a woman with an active case of genital herpes can infect her child at the time of delivery. Statistics show that in about half of these cases, the infant will be infected, and about half of those infants will die. For this reason, many women who have herpes elect to deliver by Caesarean section just to be safe.

VAGINITIS

This is a common complaint among women. Vaginitis can be caused by a variety of different organisms, which may or may not be transmitted through sexual contact. Symptoms include a vaginal discharge, itchiness, and an unpleasant odor. Medications can cure it, and treatment may last up to a month. There are, however, a number of steps that women can take in order to help prevent its occurrence:

1. Wear only cotton underpants (or at least underpants with a cotton crotch). Synthetic materials (nylon, etc.) keep moisture in and provide an ideal environment for the growth of vaginitis-causing organisms.
2. Wash the vulva and dry it thoroughly each day.
3. Never use feminine-hygiene sprays. These can irritate the vagina. If you sense that your vagina has an unusually strong or unpleasant odor, this may be an indication that you have an infection of some sort.
4. Always wipe with toilet paper from front to back, whether after urinating or after defecating. Wiping from the anus toward the vagina can transmit bacteria into the vagina, which can cause infection.
5. When pants are worn, they should be relatively loose fitting. Pants that are too tight in the crotch may cause irritation in the vulva and will also retain moisture.
6. Occasional (and only occasional) douching with a mildly acidic solution can help prevent vaginitis (use one or two tablespoons of vinegar in a quart of water).
7. Don't consume excessive amounts of sugar or carbohydrates.

OTHER STDS

Parents should be aware of a number of other STDs that can pose a serious health threat to their children.

Trichomonas vaginalis involves an infection of the vagina, although men are also susceptible to infection. For this reason partners should be treated simultaneously—otherwise, they will pass the disease back and forth between them (the "Ping-Pong" effect). About 20% of women experience trichomoniasis of the vagina during their reproductive years. In men the organism infects the urethra, prostate, and bladder but it only rarely causes symptoms, so it is more difficult to detect in men. It is especially common in women between the ages of sixteen and thirty-five. Often the only sign is a discharge with pus, though it may become painful and give off a noticeable odor. There may be pain with either urination or intercourse. Although we classify this disease as an STD, it is possible to contract it nonsexually by coming into contact with an infected person's clothing or towel.

Chlamydia are organisms related to both bacteria and viruses. It is believed that they cause much of the vaginitis in women and NGU in men; they can also lead to PID (discussed below). Treatment of this infection usually consists of an antibiotic (tetracycline, doxycycline, or azithromycin). In about 20% of people the infection returns after treatment, which must then be repeated for a longer period. If an infected person has intercourse before completing treatment, they may infect their partners. Partners should be treated simultaneously. Chlamydia infections are very widespread today, although it is difficult to measure exactly how many people are affected (chlamydia is not a reportable disease by law, although it is estimated that as many as 1 million people are affected each year).

Pelvic inflammatory disease (PID, also called *salpingitis)* is a severe infection of the female reproductive system. Usually complications arising from, or failure to treat, another STD (such as gonorrhea or chlamydia) cause the infection. This infection starts in the vagina or cervix, then moves through the uterus and up into the fallopian tubes, sometimes reaching the ovaries.

Symptoms include pain and tenderness in the lower abdomen, painful urination, vaginal discharge, out-of-cycle menstrual bleeding and/or cramps, chills, and fever. Early diagnosis and treatment with antibiotics is essential with PID: hospitalization, surgery, and even death occur in women with severe cases. Sometimes women become infertile as a result of these infections; women who use the IUD need to be especially alert to the symptoms mentioned above, as they are ten times more likely to develop PID than women who use other forms of contraception.

Venereal warts are caused by a virus. They usually develop on the genitals three to five months after initial exposure. It is important to seek treatment quickly, as venereal warts may spread or enlarge and thus require surgical removal.

Crabs, also known as pubic lice, are tiny parasites that live in the pubic hair. Itching, caused by the lice attaching themselves to the skin, is the main symptom. Treatment is available through application of a medicated shampoo prescribed by a physician. After treatment, it is important to use a complete change of clothing and linens to avoid the possibility of reinfection.

Scabies are tiny mites that burrow under the skin, usually of the inner thighs and genitals. Scabies are transmitted by genital and other types of close contact with an infected person. A small group of open sores resulting from scratching is symptomatic of scabies. The treatment of choice usually is medicated shampoo. As with lice, the sexual partner should be checked and treated at the same time to avoid reinfestation. Clothing and bedding should also be changed.

Chancroid. Symptoms include a painful sore (or sores) on the genitals, followed by pain in the crotch area. Chancroid sometimes appears together with another STD, particularly herpes or syphilis. Tetracycline or another antibiotic is the usual treatment; women especially need to be cautious, because they often show no signs of infection.

Hepatitis is a viral infection of the liver, which has symptoms of nausea, loss of appetite, fever, abdominal discomfort, and pain in the joints. Hepatitis is sexually transmitted through oral–anal contact as well as anal intercourse. Treatment consists of a carefully controlled diet and prolonged bed rest.

Several other infections are also transmitted through sexual contact with the anus and rectum. These include shigellosis, amebiasis, and giardiasis—also called "gay bowel disease." People with these infections suffer from irritation of the bowels, cramps, diarrhea, and irregular bowel movements. Physicians first diagnosed it in 1979. The risk of infection is greatest through anal sex, but it can also be contracted during oral or vaginal sex. It can be spread through bodily fluids, especially blood and semen.

AIDS is a condition in which the body's immune system stops protecting the individual against disease. This leaves the person vulnerable to cancer and various infections which the body can no longer defend against. It is believed that AIDS is caused by a virus or similar organism (not bacteria). It is, for the most part, a sexually transmitted disease. Infected mothers can infect their newborn babies!

In the United States at the outset AIDS was most prevalent among male homosexuals; over the years infected heterosexual males, females, and teenagers have become by far the largest majority. Intravenous drug users are susceptible, and some places have instituted clean-needle programs. Hemophiliacs and others receiving blood transfusions are at risk, but the blood supply is now safer. Although with new drugs and combinations of drugs, most patients are living longer, at the present, AIDS is not considered a curable disease, and much further research is needed.

PARENTS, CHILDREN AND STDS

What should parents tell their children about STDs? First, let us express our conviction that the best time to learn about STDs is before becoming sexually active. If your children are already sexually active, it becomes even more urgent that they learn how to protect themselves. STDs such as gonorrhea or NGU pass from person to person about as rapidly and easily as the common cold.

More teenagers get STDs these days than ever before. Aside from abstinence, the condom is the best means of prevention available. Various other contraceptive methods provide little or no protection, and the pill without the use of condoms tends to make women more susceptible. People can also decrease their chances of contracting STDs by first urinating and then washing their genitals with soap and water immediately after sexual relations. Some young people simply do not worry about STDs because they know that, for the most part, a cure is available. These same youngsters forget that in order to be cured, you must know that you have it in the first place. Thus we stress the value of information and open discussion of these matters between parents and children.

Parents as well as teenagers should be aware of the following signs of STDs. Parents might want their teenagers to read the following two paragraphs themselves. In general, a woman should seek medical help if she has any of the following signs:

- Burning while urinating
- A persistent sore throat
- Pain or itchiness in or around the vagina
- Any soreness or redness around the vulva or the anus
- Any sores, warts, or pimples in or near the vulva
- A discharge that is yellow, green, or otherwise discolored (a normal discharge is usually clear or milky)
- A thick discharge that looks like cottage cheese

In general, a man should seek medical help if he has any of the following signs:

- A persistent sore throat
- Burning during and shortly after urination

- Any sores, warts, or pimples on the penis or around it
- Any unusual coloring of the urine, such as urine that is reddish or very dark
- A milky or puslike discharge
- Any soreness or redness around the anus

Immediate treatment is paramount if one should contract an STD. Adolescents will be more likely to seek treatment if parents stress that the subject of STD is open for discussion. In case your child might be too embarrassed to confide in you, make him or her aware of the numerous community resources in this field. It is essential to stress that diagnosis can be made only by microscopic examination. Tell your teenage children that treatment is confidential. Local health centers, STD clinics, the county health department, the local office of Planned Parenthood, family planning clinics, hospital clinics, or your private physician are all options. Parental consent for minors is not required, and treatment is often free of charge.

There is a national, toll-free number that is an important resource for those seeking information. The STD Hotline of the Centers for Disease Control in Atlanta provides information and referrals to locally available treatment centers. The number is (800)227-8922.

There is a great deal of truth to the old adage "An ounce of prevention is worth a pound of cure." The most significant message parents can teach their children is to prevent themselves from becoming infected in the first place. Parents may not want their teenage children to engage in any form of sexual activity, but they should give their children the information necessary to protect themselves if they choose to have sex against their parents' wishes.

Of course, movies and TV shows/ads don't teach "prevention," and in much of their content they give overt and covert "messages" that sexual activity "when you feel like it" is the only way! What sponsor wants a product or a show linked to gonorrhea or chlamydia or genital warts? When is the last time anyone saw or heard the word "syphilis" on the tube? There have been some educational programs on AIDS—though almost nothing in an "entertainment" context—and we are talking about an epidemic that has spread to 47 million persons worldwide by the end of 1998. Disease, while a frightening reality of the sexual scene today, is virtually **absent** from mass media programming. We have spoken here often of the "parent's wishes"—a desire for safety, honesty, self-and-other-respect, and joy in their children's sexual behavior. What are the "media's wishes?" Well, for the most part, to sell products any way they can. In many cases sexual references, innuendo, and provocation work just fine.

Stimulation without consequences in the mass media does a disservice to society as a whole and teenagers in particular. In order to be safe from widening contagion we must practice **preventive** education! The media depends on public good will to achieve their goals, so personal letters from parents and grandparents to network executives and program producers can make a big difference! Kudos to MTV and the Kaiser Family Foundation for their innovative "Sexual Health" ad campaign.

Every male and female must be taught the responsibility to wash genital and rectal areas before and after sex contact, to reduce germs and protect the health of both partners.

Society could help reduce the incidence of STDs by promoting the notion that they are not a cause for stigma; they are simply diseases that happen to be spread by sexual contact.

By changing attitudes and putting to rest some of the social taboos that long have clouded understanding of this topic, we can help people feel more comfortable in seeking treatment. Any sexually active person can contract an STD. Many young people feel "It can't happen to me." This may be particularly true for young women, as STDs have traditionally been regarded as "male diseases." The double standard operates here. Society accepts and unintentionally encourages the notion that STDs are part of the macho, "devil-may-care" image. For adolescent girls, planning to prevent an STD suggests sexual premeditation, an idea that can seem more threatening than the possibility of infection itself.

The condom exists as a simple, convenient, reliable, inexpensive method of both birth control and prevention of STDs. When other contraceptives such as the pill, the IUD, and the diaphragm were introduced, condom use decreased. The incidence of STDs in the United States, especially among young people, has increased at the same time.

The tireless efforts of health clinics, Planned Parenthood, and other groups to educate the public have not really permeated the mainstream of American life. Television, with the exception of a very few local stations, refuses to advertise condoms. "**Sex may sell, but as for condoms, networks aren't buying.**" This was the headline that appeared in USA Today (Nov. 30, 1998). The article went on to note that ABC, NBC, CBS, FOX, WB, and UPN don't accept condom advertising.

AIDS ALERT

Every American family should request an excellent pamphlet on AIDS, distributed by the U.S. Department of Health and Human Services. It's important for parents to read it carefully and be prepared to respond to all questions—even from young children.

Responses will range from a simple explanation for the youngsters—"It's a disease that makes people very sick. There is no cure and people die from it"—to fully developed discussions with teenagers, which would include the origins of AIDS and the dangers of unsafe sex.

As responsible parents we also want to reinforce the truth. AIDS is not easily transmitted. It is not spread by casual contact in schools, at parties, in swimming pools, stores, or the workplace. You can't catch AIDS by hugging, shaking hands, or simply being near a person who is infected with the virus. No person has ever been infected with AIDS from an insect bite. And you can't catch AIDS from a toilet seat.

Raising a Child Responsibly in a Sexually Permissive World

ANOTHER WAY OF LOOKING AT STDS[*]

Danger Signs	Could Be	Complications
Common male signs:		
Discharge from penis Soreness inside penis Burning on urination Rectal irritation and pus Swelling or redness of throat Yellow discharge from penis	Gonorrhea NGU Other genital infections that also need medical attention	Untreated gonorrhea can cause sterility, arthritis, heart trouble, and blindness. Repeated infections can cause partial or complete blockage of the penis.
Common female signs:		
Gray offensive vaginal discharge Thick and profuse vaginal discharge Intense itching Painful intercourse Thick cheesy discharge Rectal irritation and pus covering feces Swelling or redness of throat Out-of-cycle stomach cramps Unusual vaginal or cervical bleeding	Gonorrhea Nonspecific vaginitis Trichonomas Monilia (yeast)	If untreated, gonorrhea can cause pelvic inflammatory disease, which resembles appendicitis. This causes severe pain, fever, sterility, arthritis, and heart trouble.
Common signs for both sexes:		
Painless sore on penis or vagina Painful sore or blisters on or around genital area Rash on hands and feet or entire body Loss of hair Small cauliflower-pink growths on or around sex organs Intense itching Flulike feeling	Syphilis Herpes virus Hepatitis Scabies Crabs Venereal warts	Untreated syphilis can cause brain and other organ damage; also paralysis, heart disease, blindness, and death. The most severe complication of herpes genitalis is is infection of the newborn during birth which can be fatal.

[*] Courtesy Florida State Department of Health and Rehabilitative Services.

Fostering a Child's Sexual Integrity in Special Situations

T*he Census Bureau estimates* that more than half of the children born in the United States will spend a substantial part of their first eighteen years in a home without one or both biological parents. Overall, 35.7 percent of all families in 1997 were married couples with children under 18. (The share was 50.8 percent in 1957.)

THE SINGLE PARENT

The ordinary problems encountered in two-parent households may become magnified when there is only one person to face them. There is an abundance of existing literature advising single parents of the unique difficulties involved, the trials of day care, financial woes, etc. The problems are not nearly as insurmountable as was once assumed, however, and in many instances a special bond develops between children and their single mother or father. One or two parents is not the issue; rather, the quality of love and care will determine the child's overall adjustment and well-being.

Single parents who worry that their children will grow up psychologically impaired should know that there is no evidence that single-parent families produce traumatized children, any more than a conventional two-parent family guarantees emotional stability. Children are amazingly resilient and resourceful. They will understandably be hurt by divorce or by the death of a parent; this is essentially a healthy response to grief. In such situations, it is most important to reassure your children that they are still loved and are in no way responsible for the absence of the other parent. Young children are apt to think, "It's my fault that Daddy died" or, "If I was good, Mommy wouldn't have left." Older children might cover up an inner sense of guilt by harboring bitter feelings: "If Dad loved me, he would have stayed." Children in these instances will not respond to vague consolation. The single parent must tell the child, in the case of divorce, that the parents did not get along. In many cases it is still a good idea to encourage the child to seek love from each parent and foster parental love of the child in spite of the divorce. The reasons for the divorce can be explained, if appropriate, but in general it's not a good idea to reveal details of sexual incompatibility or other highly personal motives. On the other hand, it is probably unwise to attempt to conceal the "other" man or woman if there is one. These facts have a way of becoming obvious over time, and inadvertently finding out about them may violate the child's sense of trust.

If the absent parent abandoned the family, suggestions that the absent parent still loves them can only confuse and upset the children. If the abandoner has lost interest or found another home, the children might be encouraged to accept the reality of it, instead of pretending for years that the parent may be coming back or "thinks of you all the time." Assurances of enduring love are called for only if they have some credibility. In general, it is best to be honest about the circumstances of single-parenthood and to encourage the children to accept them realistically.

In many instances, the single-parent home is a more desirable situation for the children than the two-parent home. If a couple has been plagued by endless battles and bitter feelings, children often fare better when the war is finally ended. The child's sexual identity will not necessarily suffer without the appropriate male or female role model. There's an abundance of role models among relatives, schoolteachers, and parents of friends.

It is to be hoped that agreeable arrangements have been worked out between ex-spouses concerning child care and visitation rights and the payment of alimony and child support. A high level of conflict typically surrounds divorce proceedings, and the children often become enmeshed in it. Parents sometimes use their children as pawns in the power struggle, playing loyalties against each other and demanding that the child choose. This is damaging to the child, whose right it is to continue to love and be loved by both parents.

Most single parents do not live with their lovers, but the majority do have ongoing relationships and/or sexual encounters. According to researcher Morton Hunt, within the first year of separation, five out of six individuals become sexually active again. The single parent can live a sexual existence and still appear responsible and stable to the children. In fact, the situation presents an opportunity to show children that "sexuality" and "responsibility" go hand in hand.

Children may at first feel somewhat threatened or jealous of the parent's interest in another partner. There may be feelings of loyalty to the parent no longer at home, or the desire to protect the parent from getting emotionally hurt in the new affair. These feelings are apt to be stronger if the child feels left out, so it's a good idea to involve the child in whatever card games, conversation, or recreation is going on. When the child begins to suspect that your feelings for this new person are important, he or she may ask if you have plans to remarry, or if your feelings for each other are serious. Children need and deserve honesty about your plans.

In the early stages of their sexual relationships, most people confine the sexual activities to times when the children are either asleep or not home, or they go to the other person's house or apartment. Our view is that unless there is a sense of continuation to the relationship, it is best not to spend the night together in the house while the children are there. It can be very difficult for the child to continually adapt to new lovers. Once a relationship becomes stable, the parent can weigh the child's needs against their own desires for more normal intimacy.

The decision is easier if the child has accepted the boyfriend or girlfriend and seems to like the person. It is often the case, in fact, that children develop deep emotional ties to these other partners and consequently suffer a sense of loss if the relationship ends. The children may welcome the camaraderie of having another person in the house and appreciate the positive effect on the parent. Sex itself thus becomes a secondary issue, and it yields in significance to other intricate considerations that come with living under the same roof. It is not uncommon for children to press the parent to marry, which of course should not be the primary influence for the parent's decision. If marriage is contemplated, it's good to know how the children feel.

In the early stages of any new relationship, it's best if the role of parent and disciplinarian remains solely with the parent. Children often resent the interference of a boyfriend or girlfriend (rightfully so) and may retort with "Leave me alone—you're not my parent." As the relationship progresses, children may welcome the advice and guidance of another adult. Some people who have no children of their own do not feel comfortable with children and have no idea how to relate to them. In an unhappy situation, the parent may be confronted with a child's ultimatum, "Either he goes or I do." It's very important to be sensitive to the child's feelings and not automatically assume he or she is just acting spoiled or selfish. The parent might respond, "I love you both differently, but I can't let you make my decisions for me. You'll always be my child no matter what happens, and I'm not sure what the future holds for my lover and me. But you and I will always love each other—and that's the difference."

When children are deprived of a second parent, they often become close to another adult—a teacher, a coach, a relative, or a Boy or Girl Scout leader. A volunteer from the Big Brothers or Big Sisters program can be very helpful. The person may adopt the role of "significant other" or may simply provide the child with a measure of closeness and friendship. It is a good idea for the single parent to encourage and support these liaisons. One-parent households sometimes have a tendency to turn inward, cutting off important interaction with the outside world. It is common that an extraordinary bond of love and closeness develops between children and parent in such circumstances, but it shouldn't be so exclusive that it becomes a stifling case of "you and me against the world."

The ongoing responsibility of sex-educating the child can be assumed by the single parent for children of both sexes. Children appreciate their own parent's candor and openness, but if the parent is too uncomfortable discussing sexual issues, perhaps a relative or close friend might be willing to fill in. Single fathers may want to seek female assistance to demonstrate how to manage a sanitary napkin before the onset of a daughter's menstruation. All other matters pertaining to sexuality can be sensitively and competently handled by single parents of either sex.

Single parents are correct in assuming that their child's sexuality and needs are no different from those in two-parent homes. The children require the same anatomical, contraceptive, behavioral, and attitudinal information that should be imparted to all youngsters. Discipline and guidance are just as crucial, and no special allowances need be made because the child has only one custodial parent.

SEXUAL HEALTH AND THE DISABLED CHILD

A while ago one of the authors was addressing a meeting of several hundred individuals who have severe disabilities, with their parents and related health professionals. After an enthusiastic half-hour presentation, the gathering remained sullen and unimpressed. The speaker had talked positively of the rights of all individuals to sexual expression and intimate relationships, and yet the audience did not respond. Finally there was an emotional outburst from one workshop leader. She shouted, "How can you say things like that when you see before you people who only have to look at themselves in the mirror to know that what you say represents empty promises of a future that is not possible for any of them!"

The answer came from a woman confined to a wheelchair. She said, "You know, when I look only at myself, I feel depressed. When I take in the world I live in, I'm impressed. When I allow God to touch me, I feel blessed."

Pandemonium broke out. The formerly unreceptive, frustrated crowd became a group of people wanting desperately to talk about their hidden aspirations, mainly in terms of their strong desires for love, companionship, and sexual expression.

Society has conspired to deny individuals with disabling conditions their inherent sexual nature. Parents, as well as institutions to which handicapped people may be confined, have responded to the rehabilitative and educational needs of the disabled in all major areas save that of sexuality. A victim of an automobile accident who is suddenly paraplegic, a child born with cerebral palsy, and others with a variety of handicapping conditions are taught how to handle the orthopedic devices, wheelchairs, prosthetics, and other special adaptations that are required. In many cases, extraordinary inventiveness has been displayed in overcoming tremendous difficulties. However, little effort has been made in the area of life that is most important to people, regardless of level of competence, physically or mentally.

Sometimes handicaps are allowed to overshadow all other areas of the person's existence. Parents of a teenager who is paralyzed from the waist down tend to assume that their child's sexual feelings are also extinguished. Families of young people who have brain injury, spinal-cord damage, are blind, deaf, etc., often make the same faulty assumptions: my child has enough to worry about without all the pressures and potential for failure associated with sex.

Most individuals with disabilities suffer from extremely low levels of self-esteem. They look into the mirror and see deformed limbs or spastic and uncontrolled body movements, and they worry, "How could anyone ever love me?" Those with mentally handicapping conditions also fear that they are unattractive to other people. Perhaps they have already failed in school, have been relegated to special classes, or have had to face the fact that they will never be able to hold a job or live a normal life. Isolated from the rest of society by physical barriers and often spending the majority of their time at home or in an institution, they see little hope for the future.

Despite the enormous difficulties they face, it is time for parents to think about their handicapped children in these terms: "Yes, we want you to love and be loved. Yes, we want you to express your sexuality in whatever ways are possible for you, and we will support your wishes to that end." Apart from the obvious difficulties their handicaps pose, the main problems these young people have are usually a lack of friends, companionship, interesting things to do, and frustration of their sexual needs. The handicap itself can emerge as a minor problem compared to their feelings of worthlessness and despair.

Information is a first and most powerful ally. For instance, being unfamiliar with the ordinary obscenities young people use can make a disabled person the brunt of coarse jokes. If you keep them in the dark about sex, discourage them from asking questions, scold them for experimenting, shame them, and deny them privacy and/or opportunities to explore mutual sexuality, they will probably suffer more than "normal" children under the same circumstances. The self-image suffers tremendously from the handicap; being denied the right to information and the freedom to express their sexuality magnifies these burdens unbearably.

The sexual needs of individuals with handicaps are no different from those of the rest of the population. Physiologically, there may be catheters to deal with, braces to be removed, or transitory sensation in their genitals. They may have to struggle out of wheelchairs or cope with shaky hands and may slur the intimate words they speak to each other. These are secondary considerations to what goes on in their hearts and minds.

Their birthright of *full* sexual expression, however, is accompanied by the same responsibilities that apply to any other person. Teenagers with disabilities are also too young and too vulnerable to experience sexual intercourse, and they must be as careful to guard against pregnancy and STD as their nonhandicapped counterparts. They must be as sensitive to other people's feelings as "normal" youngsters.

There is evidence to suggest that parents of handicapped youth spend more time than other parents in discouraging their children's masturbation. This can be an especially devastating restriction for the handicapped adolescent, who often does not have the opportunities for socializing, dating, kissing, hand holding, etc., available to other teenagers. Many institutions spend inordinate amounts of energy to guarantee that patients do not even have enough privacy to masturbate. Any person who is prohibited from exploring his or her sexuality in this way, and is made to feel guilty about it, may suffer a variety of emotional consequences. As we state unequivocally in our discussion of masturbation, it is a normal sexual expression for people of any age, provided it is voluntary and enjoyable. For people who do not have sufficient motor control to masturbate themselves, vibrators can be used with satisfying results.

Some young people with disabilities seem to masturbate a great deal, which is often a response to boredom or lack of outside interests. This is usually not a sexual problem per se. The solution, if the behavior really is excessive, is to stimulate the youngster in other ways and provide social experiences and interaction that satisfy the need for human relationships.

Fostering a Child's Sexual Integrity in Special Situations

Handicapped young people sometimes need their parents' assistance in arranging dates or finding opportunities to meet other young people. If they cannot run down the street to meet their friends, or get to high-school dances under their own steam, they will need help. Parents are usually willing to make extra efforts to get their handicapped youngsters out of the house so that their child will not miss out on valuable socializing experiences.

Sometimes a parent discourages a disabled youngster from dating or going to high-school dances or parties for fear the child will be hurt or rebuffed. That is certainly an understandable fear—yet to deny the child an opportunity to get dressed up and go out and take a chance, even to risk getting hurt and feeling heartbroken, is to deny him or her a major experience in living.

Disabled youth and adults want to socialize as much as other people. Since adolescents generally have far more social experience with members of their own sex, they tend to feel nervous and anxious about their first dating experiences. This is especially true for those with obvious physical impairments that make them feel unattractive and fear rejection. For this reason, double-dating or group activities are often preferable and easier in the beginning, as with other teens.

A young girl worried about her appearance, for example, would feel more comfortable in a mixed group. When all the girls excuse themselves for a conference in the bathroom, she could join them and share in the general concern over hairstyles and lipstick. It may give her renewed confidence to see that the other girls have just as many uncertainties as she does. To the best of their abilities, disabled adolescents can care for their own appearance—grooming, manners, and appropriate clothing. No matter how hard they try to please, some people will find them unattractive, others won't seem to care, and still others will find in them a singular beauty.

Sometimes young people with disabilities become so immersed in self-pity that they decide in advance nobody will ever love them or want to marry them. The alternative to making such grim prophecies and waiting for time to bear them out is to find or create new reasons to love and respect oneself. Positive self-regard is what counts: "If I look as if I am mightily enjoying my own company, chances are somebody else will soon be along wishing to share it."

As teenagers mature in their social relationships, they may begin to think seriously about marriage. Popular mythology notwithstanding, many disabled persons do marry and adjust quite successfully. A few prefer to remain single; others would like to marry but fear that their impairment makes them ineligible. If your child wishes to marry another disabled person, you may worry about being saddled with yet another financial burden. Parents who have already accepted permanent financial responsibility for one disabled child may find that sharing the burden with another set of parents is a relief. They can help with shopping, laundry and chauffeuring, rent, utilities, and phone bills. With new feelings of independence and new energy generated by a loving relationship, the disabled partners may become less dependent emotionally on their parents.

Adults with disabilities who want to have children may be confronted with objections from doctors and parents. In this situation, one cannot talk blithely of the right to bear offspring, or the joys of nurturance and comfort a child might bring to the couple. Romantic fantasies about parenthood abound—cuddling sweet infants while they gurgle delightedly, and loving them dearly with never a scream in the middle of the night or a medical emergency. Evaluate realistically whether the couple is able to care for a child. There are added expenses to be considered, as well as the child's need and right to be raised in a stimulating environment. Those who think they would like to have a child but aren't sure of their ability to manage might volunteer to work in a nursery or a day-care center for a while to get an idea of what is involved. It's not a foolproof precaution, but it can be instructive.

Marriage for adults with disabilities is often more successful without children, without the inevitable disruption and strain involved in child rearing. Other drawbacks include the possibility that a normal child born of mentally retarded parents may subsequently become retarded as a consequence of inferior care and insufficient stimulation during the formative years. It is difficult for even a mildly retarded couple to understand the future implications of having a child and providing years of care; more commonly, a mentally disabled husband and wife will tend to focus on the pleasures and satisfactions of the moment, at the expense of hard thinking about tomorrow's consequences and responsibilities.

In some cases voluntary sterilization (vasectomy for the male, tubal ligation for the female) may be the best answer for seriously disabled couples, for those who couldn't expect to cope with parenthood, or for those who are certain that they do not, and never will, wish to have children. Sterilization should be considered as permanent and therefore inappropriate for anyone who is uncertain about choosing a childless lifestyle.

An unplanned or unwanted pregnancy can mean exceptional hardship for the disabled, from coping with the rigors of pregnancy to caring for the child after it is born. In such cases abortion may be a solution.

Lest the foregoing appears to stress parental responsibilities at the expense of parental rights to "live a little," too, let it be understood that parents owe it to themselves and to their children to find time for their own needs. Selfless devotion is neither possible nor desirable. Guilt is no excuse for directing every bit of energy to a life other than one's own. Parents of handicapped children frequently have the notion, conscious or unconscious, that they are somehow to blame for their child's affliction. Unable to relieve themselves of such misplaced guilt, they "punish" themselves by reorganizing their lives so that the disabled child is always at the center. There are many consequences of such thinking, nearly all negative. Storybook perfection is fine for storybook people. Real children, whether disabled or not, need their mothers and fathers to know when it is time to stop sacrificing and be unafraid to say so.

SEX EDUCATION PROGRAMS FOR PERSONS WITH DISABILITIES

The basic principles that apply to a well-structured sex education program for the "normal" child apply also to the handicapped child; the goals are the same. The disabled are equally curious about "where they came from," differences between the sexes, changes at puberty, mate selection, dating, love, premarital sex, marriage, homosexual relations, masturbation, and contraception.

There are special considerations for handicapped adolescents, commensurate with their particular disability. Sex education for the retarded is best presented in simple terms with considerable repetition. For the blind, more emphasis is placed on tactility; the use of dolls with genitals is preferable to neutered dolls, and rubber models similar to those used by medical schools are available. For the deaf, a visual emphasis is most beneficial; materials with drawings of male and female anatomies, prenatal development, birth, and contraceptive information are necessary. Young adults with catheters, ostomies, braces, or other special devices must be instructed on how to adapt themselves sexually. Film presentations portraying disabled people and their need to give and receive affection are available. It should be noted that the sexuality of a handicapped person might not conform to a parent's or society's view of sex as genital contact leading to orgasm. Special people need special, creative ideas and attitudes, and it is cruel to compound their difficulties because we may not be comfortable with the fact that they are indeed able and anxious to express sensual, sexual feelings.

Here are a few messages for people who have handicaps, especially those who are feeling sorry for themselves. In our society you score no points for being disabled. Every person who has a disability has to struggle to make it.

1. Nobody can make you feel inferior without your consent.
2. If you have an interest (hobbies, work, talents, passions), someone will be interested in you.
3. If you are bored, you are boring to be with.
4. If you do not have a sense of humor, cultivate one.
5. Join an advocacy group for the handicapped.
6. Do not dwell on the meaning of life. Life is not a meaning. Life is an opportunity for any number of meaningful experiences.
7. Read. Discover as much as you can about yourself and the world. For heaven's sake, do not watch more than a couple of hours of television each day. Haven't you noticed that the more television you watch, the more exhausted you are?
8. Operate on the assumption that the so-called general public is uncomfortable with you. Most people are uncomfortable in the presence of people who have handicaps. Usually, if you tell them they do not have to feel guilty about feeling uncomfortable, they will respond.

We feel that these "rules" are the basic steps toward realizing your own goals. Nothing we have suggested is easy. In fact, all really meaningful experiences in life involve risk, hard work, and the ability to postpone momentary gratification for long-range satisfaction. If you are able to feel good about yourself, someone will feel good about you. If you feel friendly, someone will be friendly to you. If you are open to sexual expression, someone will want to be sexual with you.

Could a Famous Person's "Sex Scandal" Be a Parent's "Sex Education" Opportunity?

"*S*candal*"* comes from the Greek, to be "snared," and means to make a *terrible* mistake in your public career and "fall from grace"—*be disgraced*—fall irrevocably out of favor. With people in public life the scandalous behavior, the awful "mistake" might have to do with violence or theft come to light; in the United States, often sex is involved. Other countries have different attitudes regarding private sexual behavior. It used to be true in this country that such things would never get in the paper—never even be discussed.

Recently the chief executive officer of the United States, the president himself, was blasted in the newspaper headlines and trumpeted in opening segments of TV news reports for having made a horrible mistake in his own personal sexual behavior. He was accused of having frequent sexual contact or "oral" sexual stimulation with a young female intern working at the White House.

How does a parent deal with a daily multimedia barrage of accusations, judgments, and testimony (including the most intimate and detailed descriptions) about sexual behavior that might be totally outside the comprehension of a young child or at the outer fringes of a young teenager's sexual "world?"

If you've been an *askable* parent all along and making opportunities for your children to say what's going on with them, then you'll have no problem with this latest episode.

If not, then here's the opportunity you've been waiting for! First make an opening for questions or statements from your children so you know what they have comprehended thus far.

In this scandal (only the latest in a long list often associated with politicians, sports personalities, and other celebrities), several points can be covered. All people have sexual feelings, even the president (even priests). Once again—all *feelings* are normal. In contrast, some actions are not appropriate or moral. You can tell the difference by asking two questions: who will get hurt and what are the consequences (for the other person, family, friends, career, reputation)? You can also discuss the differences between consensual and forced sex and the gray area in between. In a recent national survey (reported in the *New York Times* by Jane Brody), 25 percent of girls who had sex said it was "voluntary but unwanted." That percentage rises with the gap in ages—i.e., when the boy is much older than the girl. The latest figures on rape are that 1 in 5 women in the United States will experience rape or attempted rape sometime in their lives, so these are very important issues to your teenager. Here are some other questions that might come up. What does it mean to tell the truth in relation to sex? Why is it important to be honest about everything in one's married relationship? Are there different degrees of honesty? Why is the act of having sex and being intimate so special? Does casual sex make it less special? How did they know they weren't risking disease?

Then there are the more graphic questions—what is oral sex, for instance? Are there different kinds?

With such a famous case, each parent has an opportunity to clearly differentiate between "accusations" and "proof"—(so often "scandals" turn out to be 90 percent "gossip" and 10 percent "truth!"). You can talk about the differences between a trial and a grand jury proceeding and a hearing such as the one held by the House Judiciary Committee.

This scandal illuminates the difference between "public" and "private" behavior. You can analyze this difference with your children from the point of view of what is private for them. (For instance, much progress has been made with sodomy laws. Whereas once most states had laws forbidding sodomy, now only eighteen do, and several more have lawsuits pending. In Minnesota a bar owner was prosecuted for oral sex with a woman in his tavern after closing time. The ACLU is now suing the prosecutor as a way of challenging the law banning anal and oral sex.) From a civics point of view, you can talk about the Fifth Amendment, the right not to incriminate yourself, and its meaning that the burden of proof lies with the prosecution. At the same time, you can talk about the need for open and honest communication in a family.

Since this scandal raises issues of varying attitudes toward sexual behaviors, it's your chance to share your own values in this area. Probably we can all agree that sexual behavior should be kind, consensual, and nonexploitive. In addition, each individual will have values they want to share about homosexuality, masturbation, contraception, abortion, etc.

Pepper Schwartz described sex in an astonishingly perceptive way in the June/July issue of the *SIECUS Report*, p. 8:

> Sexuality is messy, passionate, unclear, tentative, anxiety-producing, liberating, frightening, embarrassing, consoling, appetitive and cerebral. In other words sexuality is contradictory, it is different for different people and it is even different for the same person at different times.

There are "scandals" of one sort or another on TV just about every day! Tune in many talk shows, some sitcoms, and just about any soap opera and someone is in deep trouble for adultery, incest, rape, or homosexuality. Too frequently violence is linked to sex. Those brief "previews" of movies often contain (along with the vivid, flat-out, unrelenting murderous violence) flashes of sexual behavior that would make an ordinary ten-year-old swallow and ask a parent, "Why did they do *that*?" TV ads that blend sexual appeals with makeup or hair styling or coloring, with alcohol, with certain clothing—even with certain foods—pack enough brazen sexual "merchandising" into a half-minute to jam the consciousness of a youngster for a whole week!

"Sex education" in some form is coming at young people from a variety of sources most of the time. A high-visibility sex "scandal" can be a focus for it all. It's a wonderful opportunity to talk about one of the most valuable areas of all: **mistakes.** Nobody's perfect—we all make them. Cigarettes and alcohol are ideal comparisons for sexuality; more and more schools are instituting solid "antiaddiction" programs for middle and elementary schools, illustrating with speakers, cartoons, films, and discussions. Children need plenty of help to learn to resist being talked into behavior that could well ruin their lives. We have to teach them to deal not only with lines from peers, but also lines from sitcoms, movies, and commercials. We can assist young people to "build up a healthy immunity" against a media parade of exploitive sexuality from *Baywatch* to *Jerry Springer*, punctuated every two minutes by siren calls to find happiness by laying out $5.95.

We do it by taking advantage of every opportunity to invest in the happiness and sexual fulfillment of our children. No doubt a sense of humor will be required.

A mistake is not the end of the world. There is a difference between a mistake and high crimes and misdemeanors. This is a much easier incident to explain than the barrage of unspeakable tortures, murders, etc., that come across on the 6 o'clock news every night or are highlighted on news "magazines." And it's much easier to explain than tobacco company executives who lied to Congress about what they knew was an addictive, debilitating, even fatal substance, whose marketing targeted young people, developing countries, and minority neighborhoods. Or that we are now adding a billion people every 13 to 15 years to this over-crowded planet. All these things are light-years more difficult to explain to children (or adults). These problems need our utmost and undivided attention constantly.

Above all, we can remind our children that most people are kind and loving. That most people enjoy their families. That most people grow up healthy in their attitudes and behavior. That all people are sexual beings and occasionally make mistakes. When we tell the truth, when we cooperate to work things out, the mistakes become opportunities to learn and do better—whether it's in the area of love and intimacy, or work, family, and social, and global concerns.

The Family Is Alive and Getting Better

A new family today holds more promise than its traditional predecessor, mainly because of the influence exerted by feminism, a movement that has created a great deal of turbulence in our society. We see it as a healthy, exciting, and enriching opportunity for both men and women, one that will, in redefining family life, prevent it from self-destructing.

If there is a problem, it stems from society's resistance—from both males and females—to the legitimate demands of an increasing number of women, supported by a smaller but growing number of men. The demands are both simple and straightforward: equal opportunity in decision-making (especially about if and when to have children), career choices, and leisure-time activities, and equal pay for equal work.

The family is by no means dead. About 90 percent of all Americans eventually marry, although a majority will not do so until their middle twenties. But almost 50 percent of first marriages end in divorce or desertion. About 75 percent of these people remarry.

More than 60 percent of all women with children now work outside the home. The good old American family consisting of a working father and a mother who stays at home caring for two children accounts for only 7 percent of the total. Clearly, we need to stop placing "guilt trips" on parents who hire others to take care of their children while they go off to work. There is no credible evidence that children who grow up in day care are more disturbed than those who stay at home with a parent. Though there are many studies that imply this proposition, none has been able to document the fact that children cared for during the day by nursery schools, grandparents, etc., are harmed by the process. We know of many such situations where children have grown into healthy, mature adults. We know of many instances where the mothers never worked outside the home, yet their children didn't fare too well. It seems strange that the very people who fuss about the importance of primary parental care often have careers and make use of baby-sitters and housekeepers.

A much more ominous fact concerns the 1 million cases of child abuse in this country each year. Parents brutalize 100,000 of these children so severely that they require hospitalization. In 1996, 2600 children were murdered by their parents. Virtually all of these parents had full-time responsibility for their children.

We see violence as a tragic by-product of a family life that stresses the traditional roles of the authoritarian male and the submissive female. The frustration and anxiety generated by these forced roles often lead to family violence among spouses, and consequently the children become the innocent victims of their parents' rage.

In her book *Battered Women*, Lenore Walker stated:

Sexism is the real underbelly of human suffering. Men fight with other men to prove they are not "sissies" like women. Women show passive faces to the world while struggling to keep their lives together without letting men know how strong they are for fear of hurting their men's masculine image. And men beat women up in order to keep themselves on top of this whole messy heap. Little girls and little boys learn these sex-role expectations through early socialization. Unless we strive for equal power relations between men and women, women will continue to be victims of assaults....

The period of transition from traditional to egalitarian family through which we now are passing will exact a price. Not all men will be able to interact on an emotional level with their families, and their attempts at domestic chores may be fumbling and awkward. Not all women will be able to balance a successful career with marriage and a family. The baby-versus-career issue is an imperative one. How will women achieve equality with men in the marketplace if they choose to also have children? Betty Friedan has addressed this important question in her recent book entitled *The Second Stage.*

Many such dilemmas face women these days. Many professions to which women have gained access over the past few decades simply are not structured for those who want to take a year off to have children. Some jobs take such a heavy toll in time and energy that a woman simply cannot see her way clear to having children in the first place. A cruel choice faces women of approximately thirty-five years who have spent ten years building a career for themselves and who now are on the verge of achieving a position of status or power. They fast approach the age when it becomes less safe to bear children. Do they sacrifice children or career? On the other hand, it must be noted that a surprisingly large number of women have successfully combined full-time careers with having families. Many couples are now choosing to have "only one" and find it very fulfilling and workable for both child and parents.

As more and more women become seriously involved with their careers, the very nature of family decisions is changing. It used to be assumed (and sometimes still is) that when the male received a promotion to a better job in another city, the family moved. Now the father is more likely to ask his family if they want to move. More and more men are rejecting promotions tied to relocations if moving is contrary to the family's welfare. Today it is not unheard of for the family to move for the wife's career advancement.

Egalitarian marriage is characterized by the couple's genuine respect for each other. Equality is not at issue; equal opportunity is. Each person maintains respect for the other's qualities and imperfections, affording each partner the opportunity to develop to the fullest potential. Men are beginning to show their appreciation for this type of relationship.

Although the double standard remains a pervasive force in this country, many changes have occurred. We examined articles in the *Ladies' Home Journal* written in 1954 and compared them with articles in the same magazine published this year. Formerly, the articles concentrated on how women should make their husbands happy. The following words of advice were typical:

> Love him. Unconditionally and with devotion. You chose him. He must be wonderful. If your brain, instead of your heart, pilots your emotions, there must be regrets. You cannot trust your brain. You *can* trust your heart....You are a woman with a thousand little pockets in your being where you can tuck away little pains until tomorrow. A man hasn't got these pockets. His emotional system isn't quite as vast a labyrinth as yours. He is simpler, straighter than you are. [January 1954, p. 36]

Today one finds much more of a balance in magazine articles. Both husband and wife are shown to participate in making a marriage work. Both share in sexuality, birth control, and pleasuring. Roles and expectations are evolving. We appreciate that men are distinct from women, but remain convinced that there exist many more significant similarities than differences.

Some people want to go back to the good old days; we don't. Before 1918, women couldn't vote. Margaret Sanger was arrested for urging women to practice birth control, even as thousands died as a result of unwanted pregnancies. The patriarchal family, which often preoccupied itself with a grim struggle for survival, enslaved women. It reduced the female to a breeder and caretaker of children, a servant to her spouse, a cleaning lady, and at times a victim of the labor market. Children, in reacting to the impossible demands of being seen and not heard, not to mention slave-style child employment, often ran away from home or married early, thus effecting what they perceived as an escape. The father's dominance more often than not created a wall between him and the rest of his family.

Today's progress both in equality for women and better conception and birth control are an enormous boon to stronger families; couples can have exactly the size of family they want. The value of this achievement is difficult to overstate. Economic pressure on the family is reduced, as well as emotional tension within the family. Although much remains to be done in extending these things to everyone, opportunities for education and personal expression and constructive, loving relationships have been multiplied for both the parents and the children.

THE FATHER'S ROLE

In egalitarian marriages, everyone benefits. The woman who is a full-time housekeeper and mother welcomes her husband's contribution and does not feel threatened or consider her husband less of a man for helping out. The man who chooses to help with the children and household tasks can take great pride and satisfaction from being in a partnership that is equal and democratic. It's much more fun to love a liberated woman, as Alan Alda says. The partners are interdependent and *choose* to support each other freely. Children in such marriages grow up in an atmosphere of community spirit and perceive the relationship of their parents as

something deeply caring and whole. The open affection and communication between such parents can serve as the children's
model for their own future relationships. The children themselves
will be more likely to pitch in and help if they see that running a
household is not a burden to be tossed single-handedly onto their
mother's shoulders.

The fullest understanding of women's roles develops in those
men who choose for a time to be "househusbands." That is, they
work in the home and assume the primary responsibility for
domestic and child-rearing tasks. Enough men have chosen this
path to demonstrate the radical changes in male/female roles.

The concept of "maternal instinct" has long been held as the
rationale for women assuming the major portion of child rearing
and care. Yet research and countless testimonials from mothers, as
well as men who partake in the care of their children, illustrates
that there is no biological or gender-based parenting instinct.
Except for breast-feeding, men and women are equally capable of
raising and caring for a child.

Fathers can be involved with their infant's care from the
beginning, by participating in prepared-childbirth classes and
being present at the delivery of the child. By diapering, feeding,
and holding the infant, they form an early, primal bond. The child
becomes familiar with the father's scent and voice, the feel of his
hands and body, the texture of his clothing—all of which are different from the mother's manner of handling the baby. The
father's involvement helps the child accept and learn a variety of
stimuli and appreciate the role of a father's love. As the child
develops and matures, the father will continue to enjoy a natural,
spontaneous basis for relating to the child. Fathers who shun such
early involvement, waiting perhaps for the child's first words, first
day at school (or even graduation), generally find it difficult to
establish close ties.

The average father was until recently a passive figure in the
home environment: it has been estimated that he spent *twenty-five*

minutes a week in direct one-to-one interaction with his son or daughter. Many children reported that they grew up hardly knowing their fathers. Despite the very real demands of providing for his family, fathers should set aside a certain amount of time each day to be spent with each child. Just fifteen minutes a day alone, especially with younger children, can have a big impact on their lifelong relationships. Teenagers might prefer longer blocks of time on a less regular basis. Taking turns allowing the child to plan how the time is to be spent will complement the activities planned by the father. The father's influence in teaching, disciplining, and playing with the child will supplement and enhance the mother's role. Fathers can join their children in a wide range of experiences, from chess and checkers, political discussions and talks of sports, friends, and school, to spontaneous unstructured fun.

Fathers can take their children out for a game of catch or stickball in the backyard or the local park, interest them in other sports and hobbies they enjoy, or cook and build together. Often fathers try to involve their children in some aspect of their career, perhaps starting early to groom the child for entry into the family business. Don't expect your children to adopt your interests or career. Fathers can be as supportive of the child's own interests and aspirations as mothers can.

It is vital for children to learn that fathers, indeed all males, can be affectionate, display warmth, share their feelings and thoughts, and be loving and giving. The father can be a role model and confidant without relinquishing his disciplinary function.

During the course of these exchanges, fathers should create opportunities to discuss issues pertaining to family life, sex education, and other areas of interest to the child. It is vital for fathers to share this responsibility with their wives. Children benefit from *both* parents' perspectives. Comments such as "act like a man," "That's the way women are," and "Girls don't do things like that" are not helpful to the child. Fathers create handicaps for their daughters by sheltering them while encouraging their sons to explore. Fathers have a great opportunity to help children of both sexes develop their special capabilities and understand their sexuality in positive, self-affirming ways.

The quality of love and caring between the parents is the most significant aspect of children's sexuality education. Fathers can create numerous opportunities for teachable moments in the education of their children. Before children reach the age of five, many fathers shower with them or bathe them, using the occasions to discuss issues related to physical maturation and instill positive feelings about one's body. Many parents enjoy having their children join them in bed on weekend mornings for some playful wrestling and conversation. When children develop their own sense of privacy, they will automatically curtail these activities.

It is important for fathers to understand that silence on issues of human sexuality teaches children as much as openness does—but in a negative way. Fathers can get discussions going by talking about their childhood and adolescent feelings and experiences. What better way for a child to learn than to hear of his or her father's first experiences in love? Without revealing the sexual details of his life, a father can transmit the message that sexual feelings cross all generation gaps and enter into all lifestyles and age groups.

Around the time the child enters school, fathers often begin to fear displays of affection with both their sons and their daughters. They fear that the son will become effeminate or homosexual; they worry their daughter will develop an erotic sexual attraction for the father as the male figure in her life. Thus, the children are left bewildered and hurt at their father's withdrawal of affection, and they attribute it to something they (the child) did wrong. After a while, they may come to see it as simply being the way Dad is. The father's fears of negatively influencing the sexual development of his children are unfounded. There is no evidence to support the theory that sons with affectionate fathers become homosexuals, or that daughters will compete with the mother for the father's sexual attentions. Some girls love to flirt and play seductive games with their fathers, which is simply a way of affirming their attractiveness. Boys who enjoy their father's affections will, if anything, grow up to be less inhibited about themselves, their bodies, and their relationships with others of both sexes.

The fear of expressing warmth and physical attentions to children may also derive from the father's fear of becoming sensually or sexually stimulated. It is not uncommon to feel somewhat aroused by the wrestling and close body contact with one's children. Fathers are apt to experience warm, mildly erotic feelings similar to the ones their wives encounter when breast-feeding or holding children. These interchanges help teach children to be sensual and loving when they grow up. Fathers who feel guilty or embarrassed about those feelings mistakenly think it preferable to withhold physical intimacies from children. Fathers can relax and enjoy the love of their children. (It goes without saying that translating those erotic feelings into specifically sexual behavior is *never* warranted.)

The antifeminist movement made dire predictions: weak fathers and husbands, confused children, and unhappy mothers and wives. None of this has occurred. Fathers especially report that a huge weight has been lifted from their shoulders once they are freed of the compulsion to wear a Great Stone Face in order to be macho.

Let's examine that term "macho" and what it has come to represent. In English, it refers to a sexual bully who is domineering insensitive, tough, in order to prove his masculinity. However, in Spanish, whence the term comes, it has very different connotations. Men of all nationalities—including the Latin—have twisted the meaning around. The term originally described a man who was strong and able to handle the problems of life, poverty, and suffering. "Macho" was a family term for men who took the responsibility of being fathers and husbands seriously and were respectful and loving. Above all, the word originally meant a sense of man's own dignity (similar to the word "mensch" in Yiddish).

Raising a Child Responsibly in a Sexually Permissive World

GRANDPARENTS

One thing we do lament about the passing of the traditional family is the disconnection of the elderly from their families. As Kornhaber and Woodward write in their poignant book *Grandparents/Grandchildren: the Vital Connection,* "Every time a child is born, a grandparent is born too." We share their belief that grandparents' ongoing interaction with families is a vital part of family life. In fact, many family therapists, Jay Haley, Carl Whitaker, and Salvador Minuchin among them, actively include grandparents in family therapy sessions. This multigenerational model of family functioning highlights the significance of maintaining close ties among all members.

As secondary caretakers of their children's children, grandparents have a wealth of love and experience to offer. They usually want to be responsive to the parents' rules and guidelines and not to impinge on their authority. Grandparents may get into trouble when they convey certain values and attitudes the parents do not share or give them things and privileges not allowed at home. It is important to respect the parents' own boundaries of strictness or permissiveness. If you keep the lines of communication open with your children, all of these situations can be worked out; young children learn early that there are different rules at home, school, the opera, and grandma's house.

Many readers of this book probably have at least one grandparent still living, and their children almost certainly have one or more. Within families, grandparents represent the most visible roots of the family's heritage and bridge to the past. Grandparents have many stories to tell of what life was like during their own childhood and young-adult years. If they were born in a foreign land, they can convey fascinating information about the country and culture from which the family springs. Their experiences and memories of the past help to put the present into a better perspective and can do much to clarify how contemporary conditions and problems have developed. An enhanced understanding of the past, as Alex Haley has shown so vividly in his book *Roots,* can lead to a fuller appreciation of the present and may help to build a healthier family unit, marked by greater love and cohesiveness.

The book by Kornhaber and Woodward surveyed three hundred grandchildren and three hundred grandparents and discovered that only about 5 percent of them enjoy regular intimate interactions with one another. The study also indicates that about 80 percent of American grandchildren see their grandparents infrequently, if at all. It reveals that grandparents often refrain from relationships with their grandchildren for fear of "meddling" with the youngsters.

Children who are estranged from their grandparents become indifferent to them, with an exaggerated sense of the distance between them. Though people live longer than ever, a dismayingly small number of grandchildren benefit from what the older people have to offer—roles as caretaker, storyteller, family historian, mentor, wizard, confidant, negotiator between parent and child. Indeed, youngsters miss the opportunity to get some idea of what it is like to be old, to prepare for the later stages of their own lives. The self-esteem of all three generations is enhanced in families that respect one another's roles and contributions.

The traditional image of grandparents is that they tend to spoil and pamper children or impart overly rigid views concerning sexuality and life in general. They may say to their own children, "We raised you well and we know what's best"; some grandparents unfortunately alienate themselves by refusing to honor the parents' wishes. Imagine, for example, that Grandma objects to masturbation. While parents maintain their values in the midst of whatever conflict of opinion arises, Grandma can be told, "Oh, well, don't say anything to the child or scold him. You know how children are—you tell them not to do something and they do it twice as much." (A bit patronizing but it works.)

While some sexual issues, and our openness to talking about them, have changed dramatically since today's grandparents were young, human sexuality itself has changed little, if at all. Today's elderly have struggled with the same problems of faith, morals, social outlook, and search for meaning and purpose as today's younger generations.

If some older people seem closed-minded on the subject of sexuality, it is not only because they were raised in more puritanical times. Even today, societal prejudices hold that to be old is to be sexless. Unlike tribal or rural societies, our modern urban society gives lip service to the values of maturity, at the same time placing the strongest possible emphasis on the joys of youth. Unfortunately, many older people accept the sexless bed that society has made for them. Not wanting to be ridiculed or feel society's disapproval, many suppress their sexual desires for fear that they might be tagged as "abnormal" or "oversexed" by their friends, neighbors, and children. Luckily, some TV programs such as *Northern Exposure* have shown lovingly etched, realistic portrayals of older people.

An older man with buoyant sexual drives is often referred to as a "dirty old man" or a lecher. Perhaps some are, but they hardly approach the proportion of lechers found among younger people. Years ago, Kinsey discovered that many older people do remain sexually active, though this fact appears to be one of society's best-kept secrets.

Our position is that sexuality is common to all age groups. People of all ages need both intimacy and emotional contacts. Older people can continue to enjoy physical relationships throughout their entire life span. One pervasive myth many old people must confront is that sexual intercourse is the *only* form of sexual activity. It is forgotten that touching, massage, holding, genital play, and other intimate expressions all constitute human sexuality! Perhaps some older persons place less emphasis on erection, lubrication, or orgasm in favor of other sexual expressions, but that hardly makes them less sexual. Furthermore, research indicates that sexual inability in older individuals is not primarily a function of physiological factors. Instead, psychological and social forces related to aging appear much more significant.

As young people treat their elders today, so *they* will be treated tomorrow. Raising a sexually responsible child means imparting respect for all stages of the life span, including one's own old age. Start young to create self-acceptance that will remain with the child into adulthood and the later years.

For the first time in history, we are beginning to notice glimmerings of the excitement, joy, and power of family life, based on the fact that couples marry not for social status, economic reasons, escape, sex, or pregnancy, but because they love each other. More and more, couples respect each other and have children only when they are able to love and care for them. They spend time having fun together. Many are beginning to discover that religion is not a burden, but an affirmation of the spirit that brings comfort, joy, and relaxation to a hectic, complex life.

We reserve our highest praise for authentic pro-family people: millions of couples who care for each other "in sickness and in health"; millions of children who are delighted by and find wisdom and strength in their parents; families who respect one another's ideas, impulses, and idiosyncrasies; families split by divorce or untimely death, who find in such events an opportunity for growth and a reaffirmation of values. Children who grow up in such families develop solid, lasting self-esteem and tend to adopt their parents' values as their own.

It's up to you—the parents—to prepare today's youth for tomorrow's family.

Recommended Reading

For Parents

SEXUALITY, SELF-ESTEEM, AND LOVE

Blum, G. and B. Blum. *Feeling Good About Yourself.* Hawaii: Feeling Good Associates. (P.O. Box S, Kealakekua, HI 96750.)

Briggs, D. C. *Your Child's Self-Esteem.* New York: Dolphin Books, 1975.

Buscaglia, L. *Living, Loving and Learning.* Thorofare, NJ: Charles B. Slack, 1982.

Calderone, M. S. and E. W. Johnson. *The Family Book About Sexuality.* Revised edition. New York: Harper & Row, 1989.

Cassell, C. *Straight From the Heart: How to Talk to Your Teenagers About Love and Sex.* New York: Simon & Schuster, 1987.

Cassell, C. *Swept Away: Why Women Fear Their Own Sexuality.* New York: Fireside Books, 1989.

Covey, S. R. *The Seven Habits of Highly Effective Families.* New York: Golden Books, 1997.

Friedan, B. *The Second Stage.* New York: Summit Books, 1981.

Fromm, E. *The Art of Loving.* New York: Bantam, 1956.

Gordon, S. *Why Love Is Not Enough.* Boston: Bob Adams, 1990.

Gordon, S. *Sex: A Topic For Conversation.* (Three videotapes for parents.) Texas: Media Projects, Inc. 5215 Homer St., Dallas TX 75206. (214) 826-3863.

Gordon, S. and C. W. Snyder. *Personal Issues in Human Sexuality.* Boston: Allyn & Bacon, 1989.

Raising a Child Responsibly in a Sexually Permissive World

Haffner, D. W. and P. Schwartz, *What I've Learned About Sex*. New York: The Berkeley Publishing Group, 1998.

Klein, M. *Your Sexual Secrets*. Berkley Press, 1990.

Leight, L. *Raising Your Child to Be Sexually Healthy*. New York: Rawson, 1988.

Masters, W. H., V. E. Johnson, and R. C. Kolodny. *Sex and Human Loving*. Boston: Little, Brown & Co., 1988. New edition.

Reiss, L. I. and M. H. Reiss, *Solving America's Sexual Crises*. New York: Prometheus, 1997.

Schiff, E., ed. *Experts Advise Parents*. New York: Delta Trade, 1987.

Strong, B., and C. DeVault, *Human Sexuality*. Mayfield, 1997.

Thompson, S. *Going All The Way*. New York: Hill & Wang, (paperback) 1996.

Wallerstein, J. S., and S. Blakeslee, *The Good Marriage*. Warner Books, 1995.

Zilbergeld, B. *Male Sexuality*. New York: Bantam, 1988.

GENERAL INTEREST

Ellis, A. *How To Stubbornly Refuse To Make Yourself Miserable About Anything—Yes, Anything*. Lyle Stuart, 1988.

Frankl, V. *Man's Search for Meaning*. New York: Touchstone, 1984.

Gordon, S., and H. Brecher. *Life Is Uncertain: Eat Dessert First*. New York: Delacorte, 1990.

Gordon, S. *Is There Anything I Can Do?* New York: Delacorte, 1996.

Gordon, T. *Family Effectiveness Training*. (Resource Books and video.) Available from Gordon Training International, 531 Stevens Avenue West, Solana Beach CA 92075-2093. (800) 359-5915.

May, R. *Love and Will*. New York: Dell, 1974.

Peck, M. S. *The Road Less Traveled*. New York: Touchstone Books, 1978.

RELIGION

Borowitz, E. B. *Choosing a Sex Ethic: A Jewish Inquiry*. New York: Schocken Books, 1969.

Gittelsohn, R. *Love, Sex and Marriage: A Jewish View*. New York: Union of American Hebrew Congregations. Revised, 1988.

Gordis, R. *Love and Sex: A Modern Jewish Perspective*. New York: Farrar, Straus and Giroux, 1978.

Keane, P. S. *Sexual Morality: A Catholic Perspective*. New York: Paulist Press, 1977.

Koznik, A., et al. *Human Sexuality: New Directions in American Catholic Thought*. New York: Paulist Press, 1977.

Appendix A: Recommended Reading

Nelson, J. B. *Embodiment: An Approach to Sexuality and Christian Theology.* Minneapolis: Augsburg Publishing House, 1978.

Spong, S. S. *Rescuing the Bible From Fundamentalism.* New York: Harper-Collins, 1992.

Sullivan, S. K. and M. A. Kawiak. *Parents Talk Love: The Catholic Family Handbook About Sexuality.* Mahwah, NJ: Paulist Press, 1985 (Revised Bantam paperback, 1988).

HOMOSEXUALITY

Fairchild, B., and N. Hayward. *Now That You Know: What Every Parent Should Know About Homosexuality.* New York: Harcourt Brace Jovanovich, 1979.

Hobson, L. Z. *Consenting Adult.* New York: Warner Books, 1976. (Fiction based on real-life occurrence.)

McNaught, B. *On Being Gay.* New York: St. Martin's Press, 1988.

McNaught, B. *Now That I'm Out, What Do I Do?* New York: St. Martin's Press, 1998.

McNeill, J. J. *The Church and the Homosexual.* New York: Pocket Books, revised, 1988.

Silverstein, C. *A Family Matter.* New York: McGraw-Hill, 1977.

Sullivan, A. *Love Undetectable: Notes on Friendship, Sex and Survival.* New York: Alfred A. Knopf, Inc., 1998.

DISABILITIES

Ayrault, E. W. *Sex, Love and the Physically Handicapped.* New York: Continuum, 1981.

Buscaglia, L., ed. *The Disabled and Their Parents.* Thorofare, NJ: Charles B. Slack, 1983. New edition.

Dickman, I., with S. Gordon. *One Miracle at a Time: How to Get Help for a Disabled Child—Advice From Parents.* New York: Simon & Schuster, 1986.

Write for catalogue:
James Stanfield Publishing Co., P.O. Box 41058-B, Santa Barbara, CA 93140. Request books by Winifred Kempton.

Subscribe to:
Exceptional Parent, P.O. Box 2078, Marion, OH 43306-2178. (12 issues for $32.00)

BOOKS FOR TEENAGERS

Gordon, S. *Seduction Lines Heard 'Round the World.* Buffalo, NY: Prometheus, 1987.

Gordon, S. *Facts About Sex for Today's Youth,* 3rd edition. Buffalo, NY: Prometheus, 1983.

Gordon, S. *When Living Hurts.* New York: Dell, 1989.

Gordon, S. *The Teenage Survival Book.* New York: Times Books. Revised, 1985.

BOOKS FOR CHILDREN

These are all available from Prometheus Books, 59 John Glenn Drive, Amherst NY 14228-2197. Toll-free (800) 421-0351:

Gordon, S. *All Families Are Different,* Prometheus, 2000.

Gordon, S. *Girls Are Girls, And Boys Are Boys: So What's the Difference?* (ages 8–12), paperback.

Gordon, S. and J. Gordon. *Did the Sun Shine Before You Were Born?* (ages 3–7), paperback.

Gordon, S. and J. Gordon. *A Better Safe Than Sorry Book: A Family Guide for Sexual Assault Prevention* (ages 3–9), paperback.

Haffner, D. W. *From Diapers to Dating,* Newmarket, 1999.

Resources

Alan Guttmacher Institute
120 Wall Street
New York, New York 10005
Tel.: (212)248-1111
Fax: (212)248-1951
E-mail: info@agi-usa.org; buvit@agi-usa.org
Web site: http://www.agi-usa.org

The California Wellness Foundation (Teenage Pregnancy Prevention
Initiative)
6320 Canoga Ave., Suite 1700
Woodland Hills, CA 91367
Phone: (818)593-6600

Girls Inc., Growing Together and Will Power/Won't Power (have proved
effective in delaying sexual activity among young girls)
For details contact: Girls, Inc. at (212) 509-2000

Gordon Training International
531 Stevens Avenue
Solana Beach, CA 92075
(800) 359-5915
Fax: (619) 481-8125

Raising a Child Responsibly in a Sexually Permissive World

E-mail: gordontrng@null.net
Web site: http://www.gordontraining.com

The National Campaign to Prevent Teen Pregnancy
2100 M Street, N.W., Suite 300
Washington, D.C. 20037

Parents Anonymous
675 W. Foothill Blvd., Ste. 220
Claremont, CA 91711-3416
Phone: (909)621-6184

Parents and Families of Lesbians and Gays (PFLAG)
1101 14th St., N.W., Ste. 1030
Washington, D.C. 20005
Phone: (202)638-4200
Fax: (202)638-0243

Planned Parenthood Federation of America, Inc.
810 Seventh Ave.
New York, New York 10019
E-mail: communications@ppfa.org
Fax: (212)261-4560
Web site: http://www.plannedparenthood.org

Sexuality Information and Education Council of the United States
(SIECUS)
130 West 42nd St., Suite 350
New York, NY 10036-7802
Phone: (212)819-9770
Fax: (212)819-9776
Web site: http://www.siecus.org
E-mail: medwords@siecus.org

I N D E X

Pornography, 26–27, 46
  parents' questions about, 153–157
Preferences, sexual. *See* Sexual
  orientation
Pregnancy
  intercourse during, 180–181
  teenage, 107, 111–112
  without intercourse, 181
Preschool/preteen years, 77–98
Privacy, 217
  teaching concept of, 42, 45, 50

Q

Questions
  about morality, 216
  of adolescents, 49–50, 100–101,
  of children under six, 84, 90–92
  of parents, 43–51, 125–159
  of preteens, 93–96
  of young adults, 161–183

R

Religion, 5–6
  lust and, 158–159
Religious Values and Peak Experiences
  (Maslow), 6
Repression, of sexuality, 30–31
Roosevelt, Eleanor, 108
Rules. *See* Discipline
Runaways, 116

S

Salt Lake City, Utah, 72
Scabies, 194
Scandal, talking about, 215–219
Scandinavia, 62–64
Schlesinger, Arthur, Jr., 9
Schools. *See* Sexuality education, in
  schools
Schwab, Rabbi Marvin, 128
Schwartz, Pepper, 217

Second Stage, The (Friedan), 223
Secular humanism, 61–62
Self-acceptance, 163–164
Self-esteem, 9–10
  definition of, 11
  fostering in children, 13–19
  indicators of, 14
  morality and, 19–20
Selye, Hans, 14
Sex for Christians (Smedes), 159
Sexual intercourse, 28
  adolescents and, 50–51, 55,
    99–100, 104–105, 114–115,
    164–166
  child's witnessing of, 42
  first, 35, 130–131, 169
  during pregnancy, 180–181
  pregnancy without, 181
Sexual Morality: A Catholic Perspective
  (Keane), 134
Sexual orientation, 24
  fear of others', 33–34
  see also Homosexuality
Sexual revolution, 1–11
Sexuality
  coming to terms with, 21–35
  morality and, 34–35
  repression of, 30–31
Sexuality education
  for disabled youth, 212–213
  morality and, 57–58, 69–76
  parents and, 6–8, 10, 37–51, 58–59,
    65, 68, 228
  preschool and preteen, 77–98
  in schools, 4, 51, 100
    importance of, 53–60, 67–68
    opposition to, 61–67, 75
    principles for, 57–58, 60–61
    supporters of, 53–54, 55–56
    in Sweden, 62–64
  value of, 39
Shigellosis, 195